D1290163

"There is nothing more I can do!"

"There Is Nothing More I Can Do!"

An introduction to the ethics of palliative care

David Jeffrey

with a Foreword by Dr. K.C. Calman

Patten Press in association with the Lisa Sainsbury
Foundation
1993

Dedicated to Pru

```
W
50
J46t
1993
```

© The Lisa Sainsbury Foundation 1993

© Cover image: AIRSPACE Carole Page 1990

ISBN 1 872229 11 5

Photography Bob Berry

Typesetting & graphic illustration in-house at The Patten Press

Printed and bound in Great Britain by The Cromwell Press, Broughton Gifford, Melksham, Wiltshire

Table of Contents

Foreword

In all issues of health care, ethical and moral problems are seen to be of increasing importance. In palliative care they have always been viewed in this way, and indeed have been central to the whole philosophy of the care provided. The issues which are raised, such as the quality of life and patient choice are major problems, and have been widely debated. But, the whole subject of values in palliative care is much more than this, extending to issues related to communication, personal beliefs and attitudes and our concern for others. Compassion is not a passive word, but an active one.

To understand that background to these concerns does require a discussion of basic ethical principles and how they relate to everyday clinical practice. Ethics is a practicable discipline, which must be able to take principles and make them applicable to real problems. Within this there needs to be a recognition that sometimes principles are conflicting, as could easily happen when the autonomy of an individual is at odds with the utility which might be gained by a community.

It is also clear that the purpose of understanding principles is to allow the individual doctor, nurse, priest or other health care worker to more readily analyse his or her own thoughts and to clarify the particular position taken. In almost all instances the problem will be reduced to one of uncertainty, and the needs to make judgements based on inadequate evidence. After all if the outcome could be predicted with certainty then determining the course of action would be much easier.

Central to this discussion are two important features. The first is that the patient is the key to decision making. The patient is the focus of all the action, and must have the opportunity to participate fully. The second feature is the recognition that palliative care (as in all other branches of health care) requires that a team approach is necessary to deliver the highest quality of service. This in turn requires the recognition and acknowledgement of the range of skills required to care for this group of patients. Further it must be recognised that within any team there may be differences of view on areas of clinical uncertainty. For this reason subjects, such as those discussed in this book must be openly raised within the team and opportunities given for all concerned to take part in the dialogue. Equally when decisions are made (and the patient should be part of this) the team as a whole must see the issue through.

Some years ago I wrote a short article entitled 'Memories'. Its general message was that for patients, families and staff, it was the memories of the care provided which lingered for a very long time after the episode of care had been completed. Further, my contention was that such memories were very specific to the individual, and that they were often related to matters of detail. For this reason I concluded that it was essential that care be provided with great attention to small issues, as well as the large ones. And so it is in relation to ethical problems surrounding palliative care.

When in the introduction to this book the statement is put 'There is nothing more I can do', an important question is begged. The book itself goes on to demonstrate that there is so much that we can do to offer help and care for those who are seriously ill. It covers a wide range of topics and it will be of great help in encouraging discussion and debate on this important subject. This book contains lessons for all branches and aspects of health care.

Dr. Kenneth C. Calman

MD, PhD, FRCS (Glas.,Edin.), FRCP (Lond.,Edin.), FRCGP, FRCR, MFCM, FRSE

Chief Medical Officer (England)

Introduction

When the stated goal for a patient is cure, professionals have greater confidence in their capacities to work toward that goal. However, when the diagnosis and prognosis of a patient's illness is uncertain, or thought to be incurable, then doctors, nurses and their colleagues may become less assured of their skills and roles. The transition from a curative to a palliative approach to care can be fraught with uncertainty. The doctor or nurse may feel and even say, "There is nothing more I can do." (Slevin, M.L. 1992). There is, however, more we can do for and with patients and their families at this critical time.

Over the past twenty years the Hospice movement has developed efficient methods of pain and symptom control. These advances in palliative care have occurred in the context of what is termed a 'holistic' approach, looking after the person in the setting of his background and society, i.e., the whole person. With advances in medical technology, the public have come to expect that the medical profession can postpone death almost indefinitely. These expectations have created ethical dilemmas for professional carers. Hence, now there is a need to identify the ethical issues which arise in the care of patients dying of cancer and to develop a model to assist health care professionals to deliver appropriate palliative care.

The nature of appropriate care for an individual in medical treatment changes as his condition moves from one phase of illness to the next. The fact that the transition from the curative phase to the palliative phase can be uncertain for each and every patient, generates ethical dilemmas affecting the care possibilities. For instance, when a patient presents with widespread cancer, it may be difficult to determine the origin and type of malignancy. The doctor needs to balance his urge to satisfy scientific curiosity by submitting the patient to investigations, with his duty to respect the needs and wishes of the patient.

When a patient has advanced disease, estimating the likely time of survival is difficult. Nevertheless, perhaps the most important ethical issue for this situation is the timing of the change from a curative to a palliative approach to caring. (Griffin, J., 1991) This complex clinical and moral decision is fundamental to the care of patients with advanced cancer.

The curative phase

During the curative phase of treatment there is a realistic expectation of cure or long lasting remission. The aims of treatment are those of survival, and the patient may accept harmful side-effects for the chance of cure. (Ashby, M., Stoffell, B., 1991)

The palliative phase

Palliative cancer care begins when the following criteria exist:

a) The diagnosis of cancer is established

b) Death is certain and likely in the near future

c) A curative approach to care has been abandoned. (Calman, K.C. 1984)

From curative to palliative care

When cure or complete remission are no longer realistic aims, then palliative care becomes appropriate. Such care aims to maximise quality of life and further treatments are only considered if their side effects are less harmful than the effects of the cancer itself.

The founder of the modern hospice movement, Cicely Saunders, defines the aims of palliative care thus:

'A patient should be enabled to live until he dies, at his own maximum potential, performing to the limit of his physical activity and mental capacity, with control and independence wherever possible. He should be recognised as the unique person he is and helped to live as part of his family and in other relationships with some awareness from those around of his own hopes and expectations and of what has deepest meaning for him.' (Saunders, C., 1984)

Such a statement acknowledges that patients with incurable cancer have the capacity to make choices and to value their own lives. It is by helping the patient to develop such capacities to peak performance, that doctors and nurses work to improve the patient's living and dying. In this context the care staff, along with family and friends, become 'enablers' to the dying patient.

This book begins by exploring issues of patient individuality, quality of life, and self-determination. Patients with cancer may appear physically frail and are therefore vulnerable to well-intentioned, but unwanted, medical intervention. Acknowledging that cure is no longer possible and breaking this news to the patient is difficult. An ethical model is developed by exploring the issues surrounding truth-telling and the patient's role in giving his consent to treatment.

At the individual treatment level, a doctor or nurse may feel the need to make judgements about the quality of their patient's life. On the wider scale of allocating medical resources to the care of the dying, questions about quality of living may easily become confused with judgements about the *value* of a patient's life. Though palliative care is offered in order to maximise the quality of the patient's life, he or she may nevertheless ask for help in ending it: a request for euthanasia. A case study is used to examine the ethical arguments surrounding euthanasia.

In developing appropriate palliative care, hospices have emphasised the importance of a multidisciplinary team approach, as opposed to single discipline responsibilities for different 'sectors' of care. A team approach also raises ethical issues covering a wide range of topics which include confidentiality, truth-telling, and the provision of effective and coordinated care for the patient. Clinical and ethical decisions are necessarily interrelated but at times may seem to conflict. There is a risk that medical decision-making can occur without reference to its ethical component. This book aims to clarify these ethical issues.

Patients with advanced cancer are the main subjects of this book, but the debate is applicable to patients with other life-threatening conditions, such as motor neurone disease, advanced multiple sclerosis or AIDS. The book is written for general practitioners, district nurses, hospice home care teams and other professionals involved with the care of patients at home. Nevertheless, it is hoped that it will also interest and aid medical and nursing staff in hospitals and hospices.

Acknowledgements

I wish to acknowledge and thank the patients, doctors, nurses, clergy and other members of the caring professions who have given their time to share thoughts, values and experiences. In particular I am grateful to Bobbie Farsides and Vera Darling for their wise advice, and to the Lisa Sainsbury Foundation for assistance in the sponsorship of this book. Thanks are also due to Melissa Hardie of the Patten Press, Peter and Rosemary Diamond, Chriss Spencer-Bamford, Pat Webb, Basiro Davey and the staff of St. Richard's Hospice, Worcester, for their help and encouragement. My gratitude to Caroline Icke for her secretarial and word-processing skills. And, finally my thanks to my wife Pru and sons, Craig, Ewan and Alexander for their support.

Chapter 1

'Terms' of care

The purpose of this chapter is to set out the conceptual terms from which an ethical model of palliative care arises. To do this, two major concepts which are frequently referred to throughout the book are explored: 'autonomy' and 'quality of life'. What we understand by these much used terms will affect the essential nature of the caring process as it develops for both patients and staff, and determine how it is observed and 'rated' by the wider society made up of helpers, families and friends, all of whom are potential patients themselves.

Autonomy

In expressing his autonomy an individual shapes and gives meaning to his life. But, what does this mean, and what ideas does this encompass? Philosophers offer a variety of definitions of autonomy, each broadening or narrowing the focus.

'Autonomy is the capacity to think, decide and act on the basis of such thought and decision, freely and independently.' (Gillon, R. 1985)

'Autonomy is the capacity of persons to reflect critically upon their preferences, desires and wishes and the capacity to accept or attempt to change these in the light of higher-order preferences and values. By exercising such capacity persons define their nature, give meaning and coherence to their lives and take responsibility for the kind of person they are.' (Dworkin, G. 1988)

Gillon stresses rationality combined with liberty in his definition. Dworkin believes that independence and autonomy differ, his definition emphasizing self-reflection and the capacity to accept or change coherently. I would argue that 'autonomy' is best regarded as a broad concept since narrower definitions risk excluding elements useful to the larger ethical debate. In the concept of the patient's 'autonomy' explored here, for example, notions of freedom of choice, dignity, individuality, independence, responsibility, rationality and critical reflection come together. Figure 1 graphically defines this concept. Any decision that the autonomous patient may make should not ignore these issues even if the reflection ends by dismissing one or more elements as unimportant for the time.

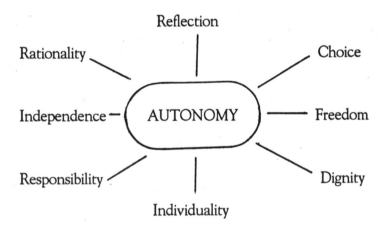

Figure 1: Autonomy

To give an example, a patient with breast cancer may autonomously choose to let her doctor decide whether she should have chemotherapy or radiotherapy, or both, if she ultimately wishes her treatment to be based on a medical judgement. Concepts of autonomy that emphasise independence may evoke an image of autonomous people as 'rugged individualists'. (Dworkin, G. *Ibid.*) But in applying the broader definition of autonomy, an individual may be a member of a team yet still retain full autonomy of reflection and action. Autonomy need not imply isolation or loneliness in making decisions. Indeed, if autonomy was inconsistent with other values such as promise-giving or loyalty, then we could not claim for it the place of most important value in the ethical model.

A differentiation should also be made between autonomy and liberty. Although the patient's autonomy may be impaired by depriving a person of his freedom, it can also be reduced in such ways that there is no loss of liberty. For example, a doctor who withholds the diagnosis of cancer from a patient, is violating the patient's autonomy, but is not affecting his liberty. The patient's autonomy is reduced because without the information about his condition he is unable to make realistic choices about the future. In a situation where death is, or is thought to be, imminent, respect for the patient's autonomy (including all of the ideas in Figure 1) is of particular importance. Therefore, in developing an ethical framework we need to establish ways both of respecting and promoting the patient's autonomy.

Respect for autonomy

Two ways of discussing the concept of autonomy emerge: a broad and a narrow approach. The broad approach works on the premise that an autonomous person is anyone older than a baby. People are free to make their own choices, provided they do not infringe the autonomy of others. People are allowed to make choices with which we as practitioners may not agree, and their choices are protected from unwanted intervention.

A narrow approach to discussing autonomy allows for the concept to be a matter of degree. The more rational or reflective the reasons for an individual's action, the more autonomous the choice. In this view, autonomy depends on acting for the 'right' reasons and people are not allowed to make mistakes. Such an approach permits and perhaps encourages intervention by 'experts' who have 'higher' reasoning capacities. The risk emerges of excluding people, possibly to the extent where only those patients who agree with their doctors, may be judged as 'autonomous'. A narrow approach faces considerable difficulties in judging the rationality of the patient's choices and in selecting 'experts'.

The broad approach also encounters difficulties. For example, when a patient's rationality is temporarily reduced (through the use of drugs or in cases of extreme distress), there is a problem in defining the amount of rationality a patient needs to possess before he is respected as an autonomous individual. Nevertheless, the broad approach discourages intervention by doctors unless such intervention is of an educative rather than a prescriptive nature. A broad approach to autonomy encourages patients to make their own decisions and to exercise this final opportunity to control their own lives.

BROAD APPROACH	NARROW APPROACH
Inclusive	Exclusive
Patients are allowed to make mistakes	Patients not allowed to make mistakes
Acknowledges feelings	Acknowledges rationality
Medical intervention discouraged	Medical intervention encouraged
Compatible with weak paternalism	Compatible with strong paternalism

Figure 2 : Respect for Autonomy: A Broad or a Narrow Approach

It is necessary for doctors and nurses to decide which approach to autonomy they will adopt, since their choice will affect how they view medical and nursing interventions in patient care. Patients with advanced cancer may be physically weak or temporarily distressed and hence be vulnerable to intervention by authoritarian doctors and nurses. Ethical dilemmas may be generated in this conflict between patient autonomy and medical power.

9

Paternalism is a denial of autonomy, and a substitution of an individual's judgements or actions for his own good. 'Paternalism involves the interference of a patient's autonomy which is justified by referring exclusively to the welfare, good, happiness, needs, interests or values of the person being coerced.' (Dworkin, G. 1972)

A conflict may exist between a doctor's duty of beneficence, to do what is best for the patient, and of respect for the patient's autonomy. For example, a doctor who believes that a patient with advanced cancer would benefit from a course of chemotherapy by extending his life for a few weeks, may not disclose the poor prognosis to the patient for fear that he might reject the treatment. By withholding this information, the doctor is acting paternalistically. The patient is without the information which enables him to make an autonomous choice.

Doctors adopting a narrow approach to respect for autonomy may give duties of beneficence or non-maleficence (to do no harm) a higher priority and feel justified in overriding a patient's wishes. This is described as 'strong' paternalism. (Dworkin, G. *Ibid.*) This attitude contrasts with 'weak' paternalism, which occurs when doctors with a broad approach, only intervene paternalistically in situations where the patient's autonomy is temporarily reduced. An example would be when a suicidal patient with a steroid-induced psychosis is treated against his wishes. Such paternalistic intervention is justified in terms of protecting the future expression of the patient's autonomy. This 'weak' form of paternalism is justified when the patient's actions are involuntary. 'Strong' paternalism however, seeks to protect patients from their own choices even when they are voluntary.

A doctor acting with strong paternalistic intent may not offer the patient options for treatments but say to the patient, "In my experience patients with your condition choose to have surgery rather than radiotherapy." Alternatively, the patient may say "I have considered the choices but I would like to know what you feel is best on medical grounds." A doctor responding to such a request with medical advice would not be acting paternalistically.

It is doubtful whether violation of a patient's autonomy is 'doing the best' for anyone involved. The claim that a duty of 'doing no harm' is of a higher priority fails, when one considers the doctor's qualifications for weighing up the various 'harms' and 'benefits' related to the proposed course of action. Doctors may be medical experts but they are not experts in the social, spiritual or emotional aspects of the patient's life. These non-medical aspects may be of much greater significance to the patient than his illness.

Paternalists have justified their actions by claiming that patients are not capable of knowing what is best because the scientific detail of the various options for treatment are too complex to explain. This is a distancing tactic, since an important part of a doctor's skill is to enable patients to understand the various treatments by means of good communication. Paternalists seek to treat patients as children, treatment which is inappropriate for adults and can lead to patients becoming over-dependent. The paternalistic model implies that the doctor has rights to information about all aspects of a patient's life, and therefore imposes a threat not only to civil liberties but also to norms of personal privacy.

Patient autonomy is best respected by providing full, honest information and ensuring that the patient has given his consent before any medical intervention takes place. Informed patient consent thus acts as a mechanism for protecting the autonomy of the individual against paternalistic intervention.

11

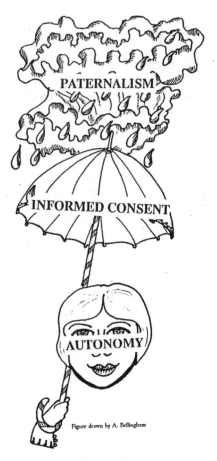

Figure 3: Autonomy and paternalism - The protective role of informed consent

Quality of life

When palliative care is being considered for a patient dying of cancer, essential factors such as 'quality of life', 'potential length of survival' and 'value of life' need close consideration in relation to the individual patient. At the same time, clinical judgements have to be made in a fair and equitable fashion so that medical resources are utilized in the best way. It is perhaps ironic that issues of cost and allocation of resources have stimulated interest in appropriate palliative care. (*The Independent*, 1991) The reluctance to switch from a curative to a palliative approach may lead to substantial resources being inappropriately committed to anticancer treatments for patients who are terminally ill. (Rees, G.J., 1991)

'Quality of life' is difficult to define because it is a dynamic concept, which changes with time, has a large subjective component and relates to many aspects of life. (Downie, R.S. et al. 1987) For most people, 'good health' is an important factor in determining the quality of living. For patients with advanced cancer, good health, in the generally accepted sense, is not possible, but other factors influence the quality of their lives. Physical factors associated with the effects of cancer such as immobility, incontinence, vomiting and pain all may impair the ability of a person to be comfortable.

Psycho-social factors, more difficult to measure, also have a major effect on the quality of life. Uncertainty and confusion due to lack of information may lead to anxiety and depression. Fears of an undignified death, as well as the 'cancer stigma' may increase the patient's feelings of isolation. Active treatments may also impair the quality of survival, for example, through mutilation by mastectomy, vomiting from radiotherapy, or hair loss from chemotherapy. Having advanced cancer may also result in losing touch with friends and acquaintances, unemployment, cessation of sexual relationships, and loss of self esteem. The patients' spiritual concerns, the meaning they give life, the value they place on their own lives, perhaps their loss of faith and religious beliefs, can also have a profound effect on 'quality of life'.

Quality of life relates both to objective features of disease and to subjective feelings, hopes and fears. The concept of 'quality of life' extends beyond a balance between the impact of a treatment and its side effects, to recognise and respect the autonomous individual - the patient - in body, mind and spirit in the context of social relationships with family and friends. In Chapter 2, approaches made to ascertain an assessment of 'quality of life' for patients are explored, together with a brief analysis of how and why 'palliative care' and its qualities are political and philosophical issues.

'Quality of life'

K.C. Calman (1984) has suggested a model in which 'quality of life' is a measure of the difference or gap, at any particular time, between the expectations of an individual and his experience of reality. This model has the advantage of taking into account the subjective aspect of the quality of life concept and allows the individual to describe his own quality of life.

Using this model, a patient has a good quality of life when his hopes are matched or fulfilled by his experience. Two ways of improving quality then emerge: by improving the patient's experience, or reducing his expectations to a level closer to reality. The latter approach of reducing expectations seems a rather negative way of approaching palliative care. Patients may have more realistic hopes than doctors imagine. Doctors can misinterpret 'hope' to mean hope of recovery but patients may simply be hopeful of relief of pain or of resolving a family quarrel. Despite deficiencies, Calman's model is useful because it emphasises the patient's involvement in quality of life assessments.

Measuring 'Quality of Life'

In patients with advanced cancer the effectiveness of a treatment is usually assessed by doctors in terms of tumour response, the percentage of patients surviving five years or the absence of objective side-effects of therapy. These are not indices of quality of life, a concept generally regarded as 'too abstract' to be quantified. (Gough, I.R. et al. 1983)

'Quality of life' research is beset with the problem of devising methods of measurement which are valid and consistent.

The question arises as to who is in the best position to attempt to measure the quality of a patient's life, the doctor or the patient (or both)? Slevin found that doctors' and patients' assessments often differ widely. (Slevin, M.L. et al. 1988) Doctors' advice to their patients is based on their own experience and knowledge, which is necessarily incomplete, and they may introduce their own value judgements. Patients, without full medical knowledge of options and attending side effects, cannot fully assess the situation. The obvious solution is that a joint assessment should be made and treatment choices must be made individually, not according to 'categories of patients'.

An assumption is sometimes made that quality and quantity of life are opposed concepts, i.e. if quality of life is good then survival will be shorter or, if survival is prolonged then quality of life must suffer. In a prospective study of 86 patients with breast cancer, it was shown that psychological and social support increased both the quality of life and the length of survival of patients. (Spiegel, D. et al. 1989) Ethical dilemmas emerge when treatments which do not improve survival and also decrease quality of life are given anyway in order to 'do something'. One example is some forms of chemotherapy treatments in advanced breast cancer. (Kearsley, J.H. 1986) By identifying such conflicts 'quality of life' studies have influenced patient care by encouraging the development of supportive services, like mastectomy counselling. (Fallowfield, L.J., Baum, M., 1989)

QALYS

The Quality Adjusted Life Year (QALY) is a measure which attempts to combine a measure of the quality of a patient's life with the length of time the patient survives. A QALY is a measure in which a year of healthy life expectancy is 1.0 and a year of unhealthy life expectancy is less than 1.0, the precise value being lower the lower the quality of life. Being dead is rated as O. If a person's quality of life is considered to be worse than being dead then a condition may have a negative QALY. On the whole beneficial health care generates positive QALYs. (Harris, J. 1987)

In their present form QALYs are of limited use in relation to patients with advanced cancer because the definition of health is in crude physical terms, ignoring the psychological and spiritual elements. QALYS fail to address the distinction between the quality of life and the value of that life, and assume that a human life is not of a fixed value but something that can change with age, ability or social status. (Harris, J. 1987) This measure ignores the fact that human beings are individuals, unique and of equal value even though just those qualities are inherent in western civilisation's philosophical and religious tradition from which springs the attempt to measure quality (for all-round benefit). The unfair discrimination in relation to cancer patients arises when groups of patients with different diseases (with different prognoses and life-threatening potentials) are compared, and then QALYS are used to determine priorities for treatments and funding.

Where health care resources are limited, i.e., everywhere, the economic aspects of care become included in any discussion of quality and quantity of life. A high priority health care activity is one where the cost per QALY is low and a low priority activity is one where cost per QALY is high. If QALYs are used to discriminate between patients in competition for scarce resources, it seems that patients with advanced cancers will always be losers compared to patients with potentially curable conditions. Moreover, there is a risk that philosophical discussion with the patient, aiming to uncover what ought to be done becomes merely a cost-benefit calculation.

Because QALYs work with averages and generalisations, they fail to take account of patients who wish to live longer despite suffering and who may value their lives differently from those who paternalistically impose QALYs. Even if QALYs were used to select the 'best' or most appropriate treatment for cancer patients they fail in this. Accepting the QALY concept involves accepting the generalisation that 'given the chance, a person would prefer a shorter healthier life to a longer period of survival in a state of severe discomfort.' (Harris, J., 1987) However, patients may well wish to 'clutch at straws' and even if there is suffering, life may be valued. (Slevin, M.L. et al. 1990) This type of measure tends also to sacrifice the aged and those who are no longer considered curable. The patient's autonomous desire to live, the value placed on the future, and the potential importance of completing unfinished business are ignored. Giving appropriate treatments to relieve symptoms in these situations reflects a respect for the patient's autonomy. (Brett, A.S., 1988)

Uncertainty plays an important part in cancer care. QALYs however, promote a myth that it is possible to be certain of treatment outcomes within specified periods of time. This measure is an expression of the attempt to justify the sacrifice of some for the good of the majority and highlights the discriminating force of utilitarianism. (Mooney, G. 1989) On an individual level, however QALYs may be useful in making implicit priorities explicit and so encourage vigorous thinking and debate about patient's wishes.

Political dimensions of health care

The use of QALYs remind us that health care resources are limited by government policies, and this fact introduces the topic of palliative care measures as part of the larger political arena in health care. Government policy on health expenditures necessitates some form of rationing of limited resources to meet the health needs of the population.

If appropriate care is to be determined on an individual basis then doctors must carefully examine their attitudes to rationing of resources. Tensions emerge between doctors' duty of doing the best for the individual, and their responsibility to deliver appropriate care for all patients. Inevitably conflicts arise between clinical freedom and the doctor's own autonomous nature as a practitioner in the health system. Doctors may regard any constraint on their clinical decisions as an infringement of this autonomy, but the autonomy of a particular group, e.g. doctors, may be justifiably limited, if respecting it involves unjust infringement of the autonomy of another particular group, e.g., patients without treatment.

Uncertainty, prejudice, professional pride or paternalism may distort the doctor's presentation of choices of treatment available to the patient. Patient 'needs' may be difficult to quantify. Some physical needs may be measurable but psycho-social and spiritual needs are subjective and involve a value judgement by the doctor. (Stoll, B., 1990)

The pattern of care given to a patient may well be based on the doctor's attitudes and beliefs, a patient with advanced breast cancer may receive very different treatment depending upon whether the referral is to an oncologist or a hospice team. At present doctors ration patient care by limiting the time they give to patients and by placing patients in a queue for treatment. Rationing has become absorbed into the 'clinical judgement', is implicit, and is not generally regarded by doctors as a threat to their clinical freedoms. Nevertheless, recent government proposals to make rationing of health care resources explicit by allowing doctors to hold and be responsible for their own budgets, has met with opposition from the medical profession. Since each human life is of equal value under the law, the doctor has no intuitive or theoretical basis for choosing one person against another.

In the United States, an experiment has been conducted in which public debate has been used as the basis for rationing of restricted resources. (Klein, R. 1991) If such a debate is to be informed, then we need measures of the outcome and of the quality of palliative care offered to patients, related to the needs of the patients and the resources available.

At an individual level, medical professionals should be careful not to raise patient expectations of personalised holistic care to a level which they cannot meet. Society should accept the responsibility for determining the overall priority of health care amongst other competing areas such as defence or education. But, if individual patient autonomy is to be protected, then doctors, rather than health service managers should act as patient advocates, taking responsibility and active steps in allocation of resources. The concept of clinical freedom, as it is generally understood, should be enlarged to make doctors accountable not just to themselves but to colleagues, patients and society.

Some form of self-regulation is the best way for doctors to protect the best elements of clinical freedom. The medical profession will then be able to act as their patients' advocate within the limits allowed by society's allocation of resources. (Daniels, N. 1986) To leave all distribution of health care to public opinion would not lead to a more just provision of resources. (Lamb, D. 1990) Consumer demand for expensive high technology and lobbying of the media by pressure groups and special causes can distort health care provisions, leaving vulnerable groups, such as patients with advanced cancer, with inadequate care. Clinical freedom should be fostered and encouraged, a concept which combines a doctor's duty of beneficence with a professional responsibility which is informed and guided by society's views of a just distribution of limited resources.

The Quality of Dying

It is important to consider to what extent the holistic aims of palliative care can be achieved. Inappropriate treatments need to be stopped when cure is no longer possible. Some treatments carried out are not in a patient's best interest. For example, in a study of patients with breast cancer receiving chemotherapy, 42 per cent of those having single chemotherapy had side effects severe enough to interfere with their life-style. Whilst of those receiving multiple drug therapy 79 per cent experienced side effects and 29 per cent described the treatment as 'unbearable'. (Palmer, B. V. et al., 1980)

The existence of substantial side effects of a particular treatment should make doctors wary of advising such treatment when there is little chance of improved survival. It is important to ensure that the patient also fully understands the possible risk of such treatments. Chemotherapy is often given with palliative intent and therefore it is incumbent upon us to assess the effects of chemotherapy on quality of life, recording whether it actually does relieve the symptoms. There is a widespread tendency to underestimate the toxicity of treatment. (Kearsley, J., 1986) Chemotherapy is sometimes used as a way of 'offering hope' in an otherwise desperate situation'. (Brett, A.S. 1988) Since this form of treatment carries such a risk of toxicity, and does little to meet the patient's real needs, its use should be abandoned on this basis.

Appropriate palliative care planning allows the patient to choose whether or not care should take place at home or in hospital. One of the most important decisions for terminally ill patients is where they wish to die. In a study of 94 patients it was found that 58 per cent wanted to die at home, 20 per cent in hospital, 20 per cent in a hospice and 2 per cent elsewhere. (Townsend, J., et al., 1990) Of patients who died at home 94 per cent had expressed a preference for this, but of those dying in hospital 69 per cent had stated an alternative preference. Townsend

21

concluded that with only a limited increase in community care, 50 per cent more patients with cancer could be enabled to die at home, as they, and their carers wished. It seems that while 'good health' is an objective of the state, a 'good death' is not a high priority. (Ford, G.R. et al., 1978)

Domicillary hospice services are an economic alternative to inpatient hospital care, so direction of resources to these services would seem to be appropriate. Many patients and their families do not have access to such support. (Rees, 1985) In areas where such teams exist, they rarely have NHS funding and rely entirely on charitable support. Patients are often brought from home to hospital out-patient departments by ambulance for a three minute 'morale boost' by a doctor they may never have seen before. (Rees, 1985) Care of such patients would be better delivered by the general practitioner and district nurse with support from a specialist hospice home care sister, in the comfort and security of the patient's home. If 'morale boosting' is judged to be necessary it would be better for the patient to attend a Day Hospice for diversional therapy, social contacts, or for nursing and medical supervision.

Some patients wish to choose alternative models of appropriate care rather than, or in addition to, the conventional treatments offered in the NHS. Often patients are attracted to alternative therapies which reflect an emphasis on personal responsibility, control, diets and giving time for counselling, information and advice. (Cassileth, B.R. et al., 1984) These alternative therapies commonly focus on treatments involving simple explanations, having no side effects, which may be carried out at home and which involve both the patient and the family.

Dying patients need a holistic, individual approach to care if their quality of life is to be enhanced. (Hinton, J., 1979) A patient writes,

'patients want to be able to trust doctors. We need drugs for symptom control. We want to remain clear-headed to be able

*to attend to our own affairs and relate to family and friends.
We want to use our gifts and talents to the end. We want to
be treated lovingly, knowing we may become unloveable. Most
of all we would like to die at home in our own surroundings and
hope that we will still have friends there when we do.'* (Jolley,
M.G., 1988)

There has been no complete economic evaluation of the
costs of providing palliative care services, in hospital or the
community in any controlled study. There have been no
analyses of the comparative benefits in terms of both
quality and quantity of life. (Griffin, J. 1991) This omission
is strange as such comparisons are plentiful in other areas
of medical care. The idea that hospitals are the best places
for patients with serious illness fails to recognise the
strength of modern primary care. Help and support to
patients and relatives needs to be offered in the early stages
of the disease, before a crisis develops. (Blyth, A.C. 1990)
The hospice approach to care can be adapted in both
hospital and community settings.

A Model of Appropriate Palliative Care

Care for the terminally ill should include the following
elements as appropriate to the individual:

a) Highly trained staff able to distinguish appropriate treatments at each stage of the individual patient's disease;

b) A joint acceptance of the appropriate change of direction
in the transition of treatment from cure to care;

c) Provision of excellent pain and symptom control;

d) Support of families and other relations;

e) Interprofessional communication directed to meeting
the needs of the patient (rather than to protect professional
boundaries);

f) Attention to psychological and spiritual causes of distress in patients and their families;

g) A committment to the education of patients, their families and professional colleagues in the principles of good palliative care.

Professionals need support for their clinical decisions regarding the cessation of inappropriate treatment, from both their colleagues and society. A multi-disciplinary National Ethics Committee could provide a lead by devising a code of practice which would have legal sanctions if doctors ignored its guidelines. Such a code of practice would protect the dying patient from inappropriate treatments whilst maximising the use of scarce resources.

Chapter 3

The Caring Partnership

Patients with cancer often present a wide range of physical and emotional problems. These may threaten to overwhelm the individual doctor or nurse who first admits the patient to care. A team of professional carers from differing disciplines and often differing backgrounds who share palliative care aims, can have the combined strength and skills to meet the various needs of the patient.

Working in multidisciplinary teams, nevertheless, has unique stresses and strains. Interprofessional rivalries, leadership difficulties, delayed decision-making, even unrealistic patient expectations are some of the problems arising from working in teams. (Fottrell, E., 1990) It is clear that interprofessional power sharing is not always simple, and inevitably this can have a detrimental effect on patient care. To be aware is to help counter some of the difficulties of working together.

When the NHS was established in 1948, the single-handed family doctor was the typical model of community care. Later in the 1960's, doctors were encouraged to work in groups. District nurses were attached to these group practices but no training was given to help doctors and nurses work together rather than in their traditional and separate ways. The doctor-district nurse team has expanded to include other professionals such as physiotherapists, social workers, health visitors and occupational therapists, forming an extended primary health care team handled through a referral system. This team has, in turn, to work alongside yet more teams, based in   hospitals, hospices and voluntary organisations. Each of these teams has its own professional 'culture' and often quite different management structures.

Successive NHS re-organisations have not made multidisciplinary working any easier. Recently some doctors have reverted to the personalised list system in an effort to provide individual continuity of care. Similarly, the nursing profession has responded with 'primary nursing' in which each hospital patient is allocated her 'primary nurse'. Such patterns of individualised care carry with them a potential for interprofessional dispute over patient management. Professional roles may overlap: it may be a night sister who is asked for spiritual advice, or a doctor who changes the bed at the patient's home. Such flexibility in roles can be beneficial for patient care, but professionals do need definition in their areas of expertise so that each understands the other's potential contribution and responsibility in care. Specialist nurses whose skills are not recognised may become demoralised and lose the skills altogether if they are not allowed to make the appropriate contribution to the patient's welfare. No individual member of the team should be seen as less significant than another in a team partnership.

The Doctor-Nurse Team

As professionals we must acknowledge the moral challenge of seeing the patient as a whole person. The sad alternative is to witness doctors and nurses directing care to maintain their inter-professional boundaries, to the neglect of the patient and the family. Respecting the autonomy of fellow professionals in different disciplines breaks down interprofessional boundaries and creates a team spirit directed to achieving the aims of palliative care.

In hospitals, consultants are generally regarded as the leaders of teams. Doctors have power and certain controls over nursing work. For better or worse, nurses tend to accept orders from doctors and maintain their traditional subservient roles. (Field, D., 1989) This outdated relationship owes something to the organisation of the nursing profession. Traditionally female, and having a strict hierarchy, nurses often find it difficult to express their autonomy when faced with a paternalistic medical profession who work within a collegiate system. Nurses may be faced with a conflict where their loyalties are divided between the doctor, patient, nurse colleagues and their nurse managers.

The vital care component of nursing work is difficult to identify and measure. It is this caring element which is vulnerable to an organisation driven by economy and efficiency. Market forces operating within the NHS have threatened the provision of the invisible components of the holistic care of dying patients. Colleges of nurse education adopting 'Project 2000' are emphasising the intellectual aspects of nursing care and the importance of a holistic approach in the nursing process. (Field, D. *Ibid.*) Nurses want to work as part of a team supporting each other and accepting individual responsibility for their decisions. If doctors and nurse managers do not respect the autonomy of nurses then these nurses will be unable to offer the highest standards of care to their patients.

It has been argued that patients require honest information in order to make autonomous choices. By the same argument, if a doctor paternalistically withholds information from a nurse, this decreases that nurse's potential for autonomy and ability to give personalised care. Sharing information within a team is a mechanism for sharing power and of respecting the autonomy of other team members.

Nurses are often emotionally closer to patients than doctors and thus more aware of the patients' needs. (Field, D. *Ibid.*) Medically defined interventions carry the risk of neglecting the social, spiritual or psychological needs of the dying patient. Specialist cancer nurses, Macmillan nurses or Hospice Home Care nurses, may act as co-ordinators of care in the community. Their role as a resource for advice to patients, families and professionals is sometimes misunderstood by members of the primary health care team. Sadly, some district nurses feel their role may be eroded by such specialist nurses and consequently do not involve these experts in the patient's care.

The Doctor-Nurse-Patient Team

The expert medical knowledge of doctors and their primary access to results of a wide range of investigations, gives them power over patients. Current concern about the extent of medical power focuses on their high technical skills and their limited abilities to communicate with patients. The doctor may be perceived as knowledgeable, competent and distant from suffering, yet with the power to prescribe, forbid, touch or even mutilate. (Girad, M. 1988). These considerable powers should only be exercised on the patient's request and with his free, informed consent. Thus, not only is informed consent a mechanism for ensuring the patient's autonomy, but also a mechanism for limiting the doctor's power. The most useful mechanism for regulating the doctor's power is perhaps the requirement to share knowledge honestly with professional colleagues and with patients.

A mitigating force for equalising power between the doctor and the patient is the employment of the nurse as the patient's advocate. Advocacy implies pleading or representing the cause of another person to the higher authorities. Most doctors and nurses regard themselves as advocates for the patient in the sense that they feel a duty of beneficence. Although in an ideal world advocacy would be unnecessary, doctors are often perceived as being 'too busy' to listen, and nurses can help by presenting the patient's view to the doctor. A further case study demonstrates how this commonly occurs.

Mr. P.

An elderly man, Mr. P., with cancer of the lung, confides to the district nurse that he is kept awake every night with terrible pain in his chest. When asked by the nurse why he has not told his general practitioner, the man replies "he is so busy, he works so hard and has so many patients, I don't want to bother him further". The nurse is aware that only weak analgesics have been prescribed and are inadequate to deal with the patient's pain. She now has the opportunity to act as the advocate for Mr. P., and ask the doctor for stronger analgesics.

This may appear a solution to the problem of the difference in power between the doctor and the patient but advocacy can create a different problem. In a team which is communicating well the nurse will feel free to pass the information about Mr. P. to the doctor and discuss suitable analgesia. Such discussion may well involve some constructive criticism of the doctor's management of the case. The doctor who is working as a team member will acknowledge the nurse's expertise and concern for the patient and view this contribution as a success for the team, not as a personal criticism of his or her own skill. Nevertheless, the scenario could be different, the advocacy may be perceived by the doctor as a threat or obstructive interference and may thus contribute to continuing team conflicts.

Many other issues - social, gender, professional training and cultural factors - can complicate patient advocacy. If members of the team respect the autonomy of the patient and of fellow professionals, then they need to share power and be willing to accept responsibility for their joint decisions. To develop such a sharing relationship is to form a partnership, not just between professional carers but also including the patients.

Partnership

General practitioners, district nurses, hospital consultants, ward sisters and other health care professionals are equal partners; they need to recognise each other's skills and roles if they are to meet the needs of patients. It should be to the needs of the individual patient that they turn, to determine who leads the team in a specific case. And, in some cases, it may be the patient himself who takes this role. Much of palliative care which is offered to patients depends on compassionate skilled nursing, so when the nursing needs of the patient predominate, it seems logical for the nurse to lead the team.

The team, made up of professionals from different disciplines must negotiate the optimal plan of care with the patient and family. This partnership preserves respect for autonomy of both patients and professionals by a process of joint decision-making and goal-setting. (Wilson-Barnett, 1989) Partnership depends upon trust and an acceptance of the patient's view as valid and important. In the everyday work situation such trust involves a recognition of the uncertain nature of palliative care in the community. Trust involves supporting the intuitive clinical skills of the team, skills which can only flourish in a secure, safe environment. Expectations of other team members must be realistic and their contributions readily acknowledged.

A trusting environment allows for open, honest discussion of views which promotes further mutual trust. This type of partnership, underpinned by the ethical principles of respect for autonomy challenges paternalism and individualised leadership by the doctor. It is illogical to treat patients as equals and to treat one's colleagues as inferiors merely because they work in another discipline. It is clear that all of the roles in palliative care are of equal importance in maintaining the quality of the patient's life at its optimum level. No one member of the partnership can do this by him or her self.

Caring

It has been argued that a holistic approach to care is a form of paternalism. Holistic care may increase patient expectations, and tends to make the patient dependent upon health carers. (Girad, M., 1988) Such arguments, however, ignore a central characteristic of caring which is the sharing of mutual respect for the autonomy of patients and professionals. Appropriate care rejects paternalism and works toward shared realistic goals. The care-giver does not necessarily have any moral advantage over the care-receiver. (Daly, M.E., 1987) The process of dying can be a period of moral development for both patient and professional.

Classical philosophical thinking on virtue offers insights into the essential moral nature of medical care. By appropriately caring for patients, members of the team simultaneously can develop their moral awareness, their character and professional maturity. Many health care professionals, lacking a formal training in ethics, have problems in articulating these notions of virtue and morality. Medical ethical jargon also can be a barrier to the communication of moral values which play such an important part in the way professionals carry out their work. 'Moral wisdom does not arise from the ability to assimilate the expert's view.' (Daly, M.E., *Ibid.*) Professional morality and wisdom are developed in the process of confronting ethical dilemmas. These dilemmas may have no 'right' answer yet demand a decision. Stresses may arise from these conflicts in the professional's moral values, leading to despair, lack of enthusiasm, loss of care and the use of distancing tactics: the syndrome of 'burnout'.

Burn-out

Burn-out is characterised by the progressive loss of idealism, energy and purpose experienced by people in the caring

31

professions. (Edelwich, J., et al., 1980) Idealistic nurses and doctors who are attracted to palliative care are particularly prone to 'burn-out'. (Nash, A. 1989) The syndrome can be caused by the ethical dilemmas over which professionals agonise to resolve. It can also result from the cumulative exposure to suffering, death and grief. (Vachon, M.L.S., 1987)

Burn-out in hospice staff has been found to be associated with long tenure, full-time status and high educational levels. Many of the stresses care-givers reported when caring for the dying were not directly related to working with the patient and family but rather to difficulties with colleagues and institutional hierarchies. (Vachon, *Ibid.*) Common causes of such stress were communication problems resulting in rivalry for patients, or the blocking of patient referral. Some hospice staff find it difficult to express anger in the calm environment of a hospice. Role conflicts and inadequacy of resources also give rise to stress amongst professional staff.

The future of teamwork

The ethical framework, which values autonomy should be widened to specifically acknowledge the respect owed to the autonomy of one's colleagues: all members of the multidisciplinary team. By promoting individualised care, respect is shown for the autonomy of the patient, and the moral awareness of the care-givers is increased. Stress and burn-out result from conflicts in our basic moral values and in the environments through which these values are worked out.

Professionals should monitor signs of stress in their colleagues and offer support when needed. Self vigilance is also necessary - to be alert to our own motives in caring for dying patients and to be aware of signs of burn-out. In discussions with hospice staff, the commonest reason given for practising palliative care was the moral challenge of the work. When death is imminent, the essential moral aspects of life and care are emphasised. The professional carer is privileged to share these moral dilemmas with the patient in a close relationship of personal trust.

Chapter 4

Breaking Bad News

Doctors and nurses are often faced with telling a patient either that he has cancer, or that his cancer is no longer curable. When that latter 'state of being' for the patient has been reached, acknowledgement needs to be made that curative measures have to be abandoned and that palliative care, to control symptoms, should begin. Research has also shown that nurses commonly face the task of informing relatives when the patient has died.(Field, D. 1989) Such intimate duties as these are sometimes described as 'breaking bad news'. We need to examine the reasons, both for the patient's fear of a diagnosis of cancer and for the professional's difficulties in communicating a poor prognosis, or a death, in an open and honest way.

Fear of death is common throughout our society. Medical advances have enabled practitioners -professional and lay-to prolong life, and at the same time have made death more difficult to accept. People react with embarrassment when death is mentioned. Those raising the subject are sometimes accused of being 'morbid' and to talk of death is considered unhealthy. Some people's reluctance to make a will may be laid down to the irrational feeling that just by talking about death we may help to bring it about. (Boston, S. 1987)

It is not simply the idea of a premature death which frightens patients, but also the likelihood - when cancer is broached in conversation - of an undignified, painful process of dying. This diagnosis makes the world unpredictable; an individual generally has a need to feel in control, and uncertainty on this scale is difficult to bear. In ordinary language 'cancer' is used as a metaphor for evil. (Sontag, S. 1979) And, the fact that some doctors may lie to patients with cancer is an indication of society's fear of it and the unwillingness to accept the notion of death. As long as cancer continues to be regarded as an 'invincible predator' which is 'obscene' and 'repugnant' then it is likely that patients will be devastated by knowledge of this diagnosis. (Ibid.)

It is of interest to contrast the behaviour of both doctors and patients with regard to the diagnosis of another life-threatening condition: severe heart disease. In this context, patients are generally fully informed of their diagnosis and options for treatment. (Field, D. 1989) Yet heart disease causes more than twice the number of cancer deaths. Cancer patients, to the contrary, are often treated less than straightforwardly. They are seen in 'oncology' clinics, told about 'growths', 'inflammation' and 'metastases', but rarely is the word 'cancer' used. The reluctance to mention its common name may well increase the patient's fears.

The Problem for Professionals

One reason why professionals find breaking bad news difficult, is that they fear the patient will blame them. (Buckman, R. 1984) Historically, the bearer of bad tidings has been identified with their delivered message. Doctors may feel guilty if there has been a delay in making the diagnosis or in instituting appropriate treatment. (Ibid.) Cancer often presents with vague symptoms such as tiredness, so time passes before specific symptoms arise which merit further investigations. Doctors who have acted in a paternalistic fashion in the earliest stages of the disease, by giving inappropriate reassurance, or refusing a patient's request for further investigations, are especially liable to be blamed for the 'bad news' which emerges at a later date. On the contrary, if the patient responds to news of advanced cancer by replying "I knew it was cancer all along", the doctor experiences a feeling of relief; the difficult moment has passed without blame. (Ibid.)

Naturally it is a temptation to shield the patient from the 'harm' that shocking news may cause by speaking about it as optimistically as possible. This desire arises from the belief that by telling the truth the patient will have no hopes for the future, and will perhaps be overwhelmed by the news. This attitude reflects fear on the part of professionals about patients showing signs of distress. The doctor may also fear the consequences of displaying personal feelings of sadness at the news. Since doctors are trained to control disease, they may experience distress when it can no longer be controlled. (Frith-Cozens, J. 1987)

Few doctors have been trained to communicate less than hopeful information. (Maguire, P. 1985) Video tape studies have shown that both doctors and nurses distance themselves from their patients' emotional and psychological problems. *(Ibid.)* A typical tactic is to assume that patients will ask for information if they want it. Nevertheless, it is known that only a minority of patients disclose their main worries spontaneously. *(Ibid.)* Another common tactic is to attempt to minimize the patient's suffering by generalisation: "Everyone gets upset when they find they have cancer. Don't worry, you will feel better soon". Necessarily, this trivialises the individual's situation. Patients need to be treated as individuals and to have their particular worries listened to and discussed in a sensitive way.

Maguire's interviews with doctors reveal several reasons for employing distancing tactics. If practitioners seek out emotional problems, they risk being overwhelmed. Uncertainty about emotional responses from the patient generates feelings of professional inadequacy, thus limiting the amount of information the doctor is willing to impart. In consequence, 'the doctor's emphasis on pain control could be the most effective distancing tactic of all.' *(Ibid.)*

Some doctors have responded by trying to standardise the 'behaviour' of cancer and talk in terms of 'five year survival rates', a concept which leaves the individual patient feeling powerless to do anything about his disease. A new myth promoted by doctors and the media is 'if we get the cancer early it can always be cured.' This tends to shift the blame onto the patient for delay in seeking advice, but can rebound on the doctor, as patients now have high expectations of even earlier diagnosis of cancer.

If staff are not trained to handle the emotions of patients and their relations, they may well feel inadequate and anxious in situations where patients actively display distress or anger. Training doctors to see death as a failure and emphasising a paternalistic model of the doctor-patient relationship makes it even harder for the doctor to share information honestly with the patient.

Medical attitudes which perceive death as a failure may be supported by the idea that every death must have a certified cause. If life must end with a specific disease it may be difficult for doctors to accept that death is a natural event which ends life. (Boston, S., 1987) These attitudes contribute to the increasing trend to isolate cancer patients in hospital for the last days or weeks of their lives. This isolation of the dying, in turn increases the fear of death by making it an unfamiliar event. (Griffin, J. 1991) Paradoxically the processes of death - dying and grief - become alienated from those who are in the best position to provide support for the patient and each other: the family, friends and professional carers in the community.

Truth-telling and the patient

If an individual feels a lump or unexpectedly loses weight, he or she may take fright. If radiotherapy or chemotherapy are necessary the natural belief will be that cancer is present even if the doctors talk about 'ulcers', inflammation or 'tumours'. (Lichter, I. 1987) In general, patients want and need information about their diagnosis and treatment. (Searle, C. 1991) 'Not being told what is wrong', is the commonest complaint that patients make about doctors. (Reynolds, M. 1978). Research shows that not only do patients wish to be fully informed, but those who are informed are more hopeful. (Cassileth, B.R. *et al.* 1980) Thus, good communication may determine the quality of both living and dying.

Surveys which ask people to state what type of care they would choose, if they had cancer, are of limited value. While healthy subjects may give honest responses, they cannot know how they would feel in facing the prospect of terminal illness. The views and treatment choices of patients with cancer are very different from those of healthy doctors, nurses and the general public. (Slevin, M., *et al.*, 1990) Alternatively, interpretation of some studies may be difficult because some patients may feel obliged to say they are happier when they are fully informed of their poor prognosis. The patient may feel the necessity for putting a brave face on the situation rather than admit to fear and depression about the future, thereby 'letting down' relatives and professional carers.

The idea that patients do not want the truth has been encouraged because patients rarely ask direct questions about diagnosis and prognosis. (Maguire, *Ibid.*) Some leave it to doctors, believing they will be told what they need to know. Others feel the doctor is too busy and questioning may indicate a lack of trust in judgements made. Patients sensitive to a doctor's embarrassment or anxiety may wish to spare further distress. But, the commonest reasons for patients not asking for information is that they are not given the time, privacy or encouragement to do so. (Lichter, 1989 and Maguire, *Ibid.*)

A minority of patients clearly have no wish to know their diagnosis. Usually this is expressed to the doctor by a statement indicating they do not want to know what the future holds, or they do not wish to be bothered with medical matters. (Lichter, I. 1987) This choice should be respected as long as the doctor is aware that the patient is free to change his mind at a later date, and gives the person the opportunity to do so. Communication is a dynamic process and a patient's need for information changes over time. It is a mistake to label patients as those who 'want to know' and those who 'do not want to know'. The level and pace of information-giving should be determined by the patient. Breaking the news then becomes a process of listening and helping the patient to discover the truth in his own way. Neverthless, information may have to be repeated, since patients rarely absorb all the news at once.

Risks and problems of truth-telling

The individual practitioner giving the bad news needs to be aware of likely responses of the patient. If prepared for a patient to be distressed, shocked or angry, the professional is better able to give support and enable an understanding of the implications of the information. The patient's initial reaction depends both upon the level of trust placed in the doctor, and the way in which the information is imparted. (Lichter, I. 1987) The patient's perception of the state of his own health before receiving the news is also important.

Mrs. A.

To give an example: Mrs. A, a middle-aged woman with advanced ovarian cancer, already treated unsuccessfully with surgery and chemotherapy, comes to the outpatient clinic with obvious weight loss and an abdomen grossly distended by tumour. She asks, "Is it serious doctor?" It seems obvious to the doctor that she is terminally ill, yet her question implies that she is still hopeful that she may not be seriously ill. The doctor needs first to discover how she really perceives her present condition, and then how much she wants to know, i.e. whether or not she is looking for bland reassurance or an honest discussion of her condition. If the doctor is satisfied that Mrs. A. wants information and then gives her the news that no further treatment can cure the cancer, she may react in several ways. She may react to this 'bad news' with denial if she is not 'ready' to receive the information. Anger may be the prominent emotion if she believes she has been deceived by other doctors and her family in the past. She may be distressed, frightened and feel the need to cry. In addition, her fears may be rationally based on personal knowledge of a friend or relative - unknown to the doctor - who had previously suffered a bad death from cancer. Positive reactions may also occur; she may be grateful to learn the truth. She may be prepared to accept that an end is in view, and being told may enable her to complete unfinished business without further doubts. Nonetheless, at different times in the remaining course of her illness, her responses to the situation may vary.

Doctors may be tempted to be truthful only to patients they believe will take the news "well". (Lichter, I., 1987) This attitude is a cause for concern, as studies also show that professionals tend to underestimate the patient's coping strategies. (Cassileth, B., *et al.* 1980).

Kubler-Ross found that most people reacted to the awareness of terminal illness with initial denial. (Kubler-Ross, E. 1970) Denial acts as a buffer against unexpected shocking news, allowing time for the patient to prepare himself. In this situation, denial acts as a useful coping mechanism. Nevertheless, the same patient may be willing to talk about the diagnosis and prognosis at a later stage. Kubler-Ross suggests that patients use denial more frequently when confronted by practitioners who also use this form of coping mechanism for their own reasons. Thus, possibly the more one is distressed by dealing with death, the more weight one gives to the damage caused by discussing it.

Mr. T.

There is a fear on the part of some practitioners that the news is so devastating that the patient may commit suicide, yet experience shows that this is a rare response. (Veatch, R. 1989). It is not so much the certainty of the bad news, but the uncertainty which patients find so difficult to bear. A striking example of this fact is the case of a sixty year old postman, Mr. T. who killed himself after having a chest X-ray. In a note left for his wife and family he told of his terrible fears of cancer. He wrote he could not bear waiting to have his fears confirmed. A few days later, the chest X-ray report showed chronic bronchitis with no evidence of cancer. Mr. T.'s case illustrates the high degree of suspicion and fear of cancer which may be much worse than the reality. The tragedy resulted not from being honest or dishonest, but from not having had enough communication with the patient at the earliest opportunity.

It is not only the patient's emotional and psychological well-being which may be affected through communication. Some evidence indicates that the way a person reacts to his cancer may influence his length of survival. (Lovestone, S. et al. 1991) Greer has shown that feelings of helplessness, hopelessness and unquestioning acceptance have an adverse effect on prognosis. (Greer, S. 1983) In this study, 'a fighting spirit' and 'denial' correlated with longer periods of remission. The responses of helplessness and hopelessness are furthered by poor communication. Thus it may be that by withholding information, far from protecting patients, doctors may be harming them.

The anxiety, distress or anger felt by patients, should be accepted as a normal reaction to the diagnosis of cancer. If these coping mechanisms are used in the short term they are likely to be followed by acceptance and adjustment in the longer term. Short-term distress is not a significant harm but a necessary prelude to longer term benefits for patients and their relations.

Chapter 5

The Patient's Need for Information

Historical records suggest that in the nineteenth century patients were generally told the truth about their illnesses, although little could be done for them. By the middle of the twentieth century, when diagnostic abilities outstripped treatment options, deception became more common. Over the last thirty years there has been a general move towards greater professional honesty in communicating with patients. (Searle, C. 1991) The change in attitudes toward the importance of communication between professionals and patients may in part be due to the impact of the hospice movement. In situations where cure is no longer possible, effective pain and symptom control can still be given, and therefore all involved feel less inadequate.

Within this trend towards more open and frank discussion, it appears that it is often the doctor's attitude to truth-telling rather than the patient's need that determines whether or not the patient is fully informed. (Lichter, I. 1987) Doctors may be seen as 'tellers' or 'non-tellers' of the truth. Either behaviour as one practitioner's 'stock response' is directed towards coping with their own fears rather than focussing on those of the individual patient.

Patients are highly likely to be left to guess for themselves that they are dying, and the emotional isolation this produces can only be guessed at in the absence of the patient's own stories.

(Searle, C. 1991)

Nowadays hospital doctors are more likely to tell patients their diagnosis. But they still experience considerable difficulty in telling patients they are dying. *(Ibid.)* A considerable problem arises when a relative rather than the patient, is first informed of the diagnosis. Due to individual circumstances this may, of course, be necessary, but the relative's instinctive reaction may be to protect the loved one by telling the doctor, 'she/he must not be told - this news could kill'. Nevertheless, this type of collusion over information often leads to a tense atmosphere, isolating patients from their families and other professional carers. The case of David illustrates.

David

David, a 50 year old bank manager was dying of lung cancer, but his wife and son insisted that he should not be told his diagnosis. Pain control was difficult because David was frightened and did not understand. Concurrently, David's wife was found to have stomach cancer. When informed, the son asked the surgeon to tell his mother it was a benign ulcer. Over time the son became depressed, withdrawn and unable to make contact with either of his parents while living in fear of their deaths. David, in his ignorance, remained anxious and in pain. As the family could not cope at home, he was admitted to hospital where he died alone. Subsequently his wife recovered from her cancer.

This sad history illustrates the cost of maintaining a deception to other members of the patient's family. The patient becomes isolated and the relatives feel guilty at a time when both need support and to be able to share their feeling for each other.

Looked at from the professional's perspective, it should be acknowledged that it is not only the patient and relations who have autonomy. The doctor should not be forced by relatives into deceiving patients. If it is given that the normal moral standard is one which upholds truth-telling, requests by relatives that a doctor should do otherwise, challenge the doctor's moral integrity. The response to this challenge should be to take time to talk to relatives, acknowledge and empathise with their distress, praise their good intentions and explain how collusion is isolating them from the patient. The consequences of maintaining deception should be gently explored: the emotional strain of keep up pretences, the likely reaction of anger which follows when the patient eventually discovers that he is dying, and the closing off of the patient's chances of completing any unfinished business of his own.

Interprofessional truth-telling

An important element in the professional response to patients' needs for information about their condition, resides outside of the doctor-patient relationship in the arena of interprofessional relationships. Doctors control the amount of information which they give not only to patients and relatives but also to nurses and other professionals. In the family model of paternalism, doctors are identified as fathers, nurses and other helpers as mothers and patients as children to be cared for. This out-dated model perpetuates the subservient role of the nurse, in the same vein as wives being subservient to their husbands.

Patients tend to talk to nurses as they are usually more accessible and are thought to have more time and duties in this direction. The nurses are fully aware that consultants often do not have the time to spend giving information or even in drawing out the individual's major concerns. Nurses wish to be honest but are also constrained by fears of overstepping the level of information already obtained and interpreted by the patient, and being reprimanded for doing so.

It is the doctor rather than the nurse who makes the diagnostic and prognostic decision to change from a curative to a palliative approach. And, this decision 'legitimates' (culturally accepts) the patient's entry into the dying process. (Field, D. 1989) Field distinguishes 'clinical death' - the absence of life signs such as respiration and heart beat - and 'social death', which is the process in which staff, relatives, and friends withdraw from the terminally ill. Collusion is major contributary factor in isolating the dying patient. The patient becomes suspicious because of bodily changes, changes in treatment, and then due to the staff's reluctance to talk about the illness. To avoid the 'social death' of a patient, open honest communication between staff and patients remains the message. A relaxed atmosphere is created. In this context, the mutual respect, trust and friendliness between doctors and nurses leads to their corporate and individual skills being employed in an optimal way. *(Ibid.)*

An ethical framework and its importance

Patients with cancer are no different from other individuals. They still require honest information to enable them to plan for the future and to enjoy the best quality of life. (Slevin, M. 1987) A patient-centred approach concentrates on this need for full information, and sets limits on doctors' perceptions and beliefs. By the willingness shown to provide practical and straightforward information, a doctor reveals respect for the patient's autonomy.

Communication (a two-way process) becomes meaningless if there is no overriding moral obligation to be truthful. In an everyday social context we would expect a stranger to be truthful if we asked for directions. (Gillon, R. 1990) The doctor-patient relationship and the interprofessional relationship is based on trust, which is threatened if one partner is found to be lying. Doctors are quick to complain, 'how can I help him if he will not tell me the truth'. If the doctor is not truthful then trust evaporates and the staff and patients are not in positions to make rational decisions on care.

The burden of justification must therefore be on the doctor who lies or withholds information from the patient, and who becomes inaccessible and insensitive to the information needs of colleagues working with that patient. It is not only the individual act of lying which is morally relevant, but the cumulative effect of such acts which lead to a public distrust of the medical profession.

It is worrying to know that doctors, whose integrity is highly valued by society, are sometimes distrusted by individual cancer patients. This is evident when some patients seem to expect that the doctor will lie, or withhold information in a paternalistic way.

The professions often justify a lie by saying that the 'truth' is not known. Though this statement is literally true, uncertainty about diagnosis, treatment or prognosis is not a valid reason for lying. Philosophical debate about the nature of truth is beyond the scope of this book, but even if the absolute truth of a situation is uncertain, the level of knowledge can still be communicated to the patient in an honest and sensitive way. A professional should appreciate the clear distinction between the philosophical concept of 'truth' and 'telling the truth', wherein his intention to respect the patient's individuality and autonomy is his prime motivation.

The argument may on occasion surface that the truth is too complex for the patient to comprehend. Nevertheless, language can be simplified so that the majority of patients can understand. Another tactic which some professionals employ to deceive themselves, is to use medical jargon, fulfilling their obligation to 'tell and talk' with the patient, but having no clear idea of the level of intelligibility and communication experienced. "The neoplasm in your breast has metastasised to your dorsal spine" may be one way of avoiding informing the patient that the cancer is progressive and that curative treatment is no longer possible.

Some doctors feel they could not lie to a patient but also feel no obligation to tell the 'whole truth', even if the patient asks. Setting aside, again, the philosophical question of whether or not there is a 'whole truth' for any individual patient or category of patients, there is little difference between an act (lying) and an omission (withholding the truth). If the patient finds knowledge of the cancer helpful in making plans for the future, withholding the information and deliberately lying have the same consequences. Accepting there is a moral duty to be truthful, is also accepting that lying is morally wrong. Withholding information is equally immoral because there is a failure to fulfill the expectations of the special relationship which exists between a doctor and a patient. Though the doctor may still argue that either lying or withholding information is justified, he cannot appeal to Acts and Omission doctrine for support. (Gillon, R. 1985)

The Hippocratic Oath says little about telling the truth although it does lay down rules about confidentiality. Perhaps Hippocrates foresaw the difficulties inherent in his paternalistic approach and wanted doctors to adopt an individualistic approach with regard to truth telling. The lesson then is that in each and every situation, the doctor must consider how his Act or Omission will affect the patient's autonomy.

Future developments

There are a number of ways in which the short term distress of having to impart what we have termed 'bad news' can be minimised. Training is needed to show doctors and nurses that emotional involvement with patients can improve their own quality of life. Trained staff need to have the confidence to explore issues with patients which they are aware will be distressing but nonetheless have to be confronted if patients are to be treated as autonomous individuals. Control of pain and other distressing symptoms, enables a patient to have more autonomy, not just in a physical sense but also in psychological, spiritual and social ways. Doctors and nurses need to improve communication skills. Courses have been developed to improve skills and are now becoming widely available. (Maguire, P. *et al.* 1988 1,2,3)

Health care teams also need to improve their interprofessional communications 'systems' and practices. Doctors need to demystify cancer and its treatment, and if staff are prepared to talk openly about 'cancer', using that term, much of the tension surrounding the breaking of this 'bad news' would disappear.

Professionals who have difficulty communicating diagnositic and prognostic 'truths' should be able to acknowledge their problems and recognise the resulting stress. They need to share their uncertainties with other members of the team who are able to provide support.

From whatever viewpoint, however, 'medicine remains the sort of job where expressions of inability to cope are viewed as weakness.' (Aitken, H. 1991) We need to make death an acceptable topic for discussion in palliative care, and in everyday life, not to trivialise it but to accept it. The challenge for medical education is to effect these changes of attitude, a more difficult task than improving knowledge of control of physical symptoms. An approach which places respect for autonomy as the highest priority of ethical health care will result in benefits, not only for the patient and his relations, but also for the professionals who will retain society's trust and confidence.

Chapter 6

Informed Consent

When a patient faces life-threatening illness, especially when his life expectancy appears to be short, it tempts doctors, motivated by an urge to help the patient, to decide what is 'best'. A strong mechanism is necessary, therefore, to protect the patient's autonomy, since this is the final opportunity for the person to exercise control over care decisions. In a situation where a cure or a prolonged remission is possible, a patient may be willing to trade some of his autonomy for long-term benefits. The individual may then accept that the 'doctor must know best'. When, however, there is no hope of cure and thus no 'long-term benefit', there should be the requirement for freely given, informed consent by the patient before any medical intervention. In the ethical model of palliative care suggested in this book, informed consent is a powerful and practical method of protecting the patient's autonomy.

Informed consent has legal, moral and practical implications in daily practice and clinical research. In clinical practice the courts review informed consent retrospectively: a patient who has suffered harm brings a case of negligence. In research, consent is dealt with by prospective guidelines which establish the need for informed consent before a clinical trial can begin. The 1947 *Nuremberg Code* was drawn up as a result of society's revulsion against Nazi experimentation on prisoners. This was a formal acknowledgement of medicine's capability to harm as well as to benefit. This code has been replaced by the 1964 *Declaration of Helsinki* which is concerned with informed consent in medical research. In palliative medicine the boundary between medical care and clinical research is not always clear. English Law tends to leave the issue of informed consent to doctors, giving them a legal responsibility for making the moral decisions. It is these ethical issues, rather than legal obligations, which are of most relevance in this analysis of informed consent.

All medical interventions whether diagnostic, therapeutic or for research, carry the potential for violating patient autonomy. The central function of informed consent is to ensure a sharing of power and knowledge between doctor and patient. Through this sharing process patients receive appropriate care from doctors in whom they trust, and doctors gain a deeper understanding of the patient's needs. Informed consent can be viewed as an expression of two elements of care: one responsive to the patient's wishes and the other protective from harmful intervention. (Baum, M. *et al.*, 1989) Informed consent is a dialogue between a patient and his doctor in which both become aware of potential harms and benefits for the patient. Informed consent is thus much more than a granting of permission.

Gillon defines informed consent as: 'a voluntary uncoerced decision, made by a sufficiently competent or autonomous person, on the basis of adequate information and deliberation, to accept rather than reject some proposed course of action that will affect him or her.' (Gillon, R. 1985) The components of this definition will be examined in some detail.

A Voluntary Uncoerced Decision

A patient should be allowed to choose to accept or reject a proposed treatment freely, without coercion. In seeking informed consent there is a danger that the distinction between coercion and persuasion may be lost. Persuasion aims to enlist the patient's co-operation by providing information. Coercion manipulates a patient's decision by influences which undermine his independent reasoning. An example of coercion would be to deny a patient follow-up care if he refused to take the doctor's advice. (Gillett, G.R., 1989) Environmental conditions, can be coercive by failing to respect the patient's privacy. There may be pressures to make decisions to prevent other patients waiting. Although consent forms are mandatory for even the simplest surgical intervention, often none are offered for medical treatments such as chemotherapy regimes, which potentially may be more harmful. Withholding relevant information can be another form of coercion. (Faulder, C. 1985) Patients may wish to reject treatment, when life expectancy is short, and doctors need very strong reasons for overriding such autonomous choices.

A Sufficiently Competent Person

A doctor responsible for informing a patient must assess the patient's competence to understand a therapy or research trial. He needs to be satisfied that the patient has the ability to weigh risks against benefits and then to make an informed decision, based on this understanding. (Beauchamp, T.L., Childress, J.E., 1983)

An unconscious patient is quite obviously incompetent to make decisions. All cases, however, are not so clear cut. If a patient is shocked or denying the diagnosis of cancer, he may be temporarily incompetent. Fear of death may temporarily reduce a patient's competence to make autonomous choices. (Farsides, C.C.S., 1989) The doctor, acting in a paternalistic fashion, may make a decision on his behalf, providing the intention is to protect the patient's future autonomy. This reasoning works if there is enough time available to expect the patient's improvement. A doctor's judgement about the patient's level of competences needs to be revised frequently, and should not rely on stereotypes or generalisations.

Care must be taken to avoid misinterpreting different ethical or cultural attitudes to illness as indicating a lack of understanding. If the patient is capable or can become capable of a level of understanding that is adequate for autonomous choices, the case for paternalistic intervention is weak. A member of the family or a nurse may be able to assist a patient to better understanding of the situation. However, below this level of comprehension, the case for paternalism becomes stronger as the principle of 'doing the best' assumes a greater priority than that of autonomy.

The assessment of a patient's decision-making capacity is an integral part of doctor-patient communication. Competence is also a legal concept, which includes: 'the skills of communicating a choice, understanding relevant information, appreciating the current situation and its consequences, and manipulating information rationally.' (Appelbaum, P.S. *et al.*, 1988) Detailed legal analysis is beyond the scope of this book. Nevertheless, it is impossible to assess a patient's competence, if he has been inadequately informed by the professional. To be able to exhibit decision-making abilities, patients must have sufficient information, and time to assimilate that information, in order to collaborate on care decisions.

A Sufficiently Autonomous Person

Patients generally want information with regard to appropriate treatments. They do not seem to want ultimate responsibility for the clinical decision. A patient with breast cancer who was entered into a clinical trial and found later that her treatment had been determined by computer randomisation, without her consent, described her feelings as follows:

'My rights to have information and to choose, and my responsibility for my own body were denied. My trust was abused. I am both deeply hurt and bitterly disappointed to have been so misused by members of the medical profession.' (Anon. 1988)

The requirement for information is an essential first step which should precede any medical intervention, if the patient is to have his autonomy respected, and the 'quality' of his life enhanced to the end. If the patient then chooses to hand over control to the doctor, this does not reduce his autonomy. (Sutherland, H.J. *et al.*, 1989)

One potential difficulty with giving patients total responsibility for the treatment choice, can be that they then also assume responsibility for the outcome of the treatment chosen. If the treatment in the individual case proves unsuccessful then the person may experience emotional distress for having chosen 'wrongly'. In a study of 60 cancer patients, it was found that patients preferred a pattern of shared decision-making with their doctors. (Degner, L. *et al.*, 1988) The amount of control a patient wishes to exert varies between giving all power to the doctor at one extreme, and retaining all control himself at the other.

Adequate Information and Deliberation

Unfortunately, there is a discrepancy between the ideal of informed consent and its practice. A study of 200 cancer patients showed that only 60 per cent of patients understood the nature of their proposed treatment, while only 40 per cent of them had read the consent form 'carefully'. (Cassileth, B.R. *et al.*, 1980) Most patients believed that consent forms were a legal requirement to protect the rights of the doctor, or that they would not receive the necessary treatment unless the form was signed. The process of informed consent has nothing to do with the practice of hastily collecting patient's signatures before going to surgical theatre for operations.

Bed-ridden patients are less able to recall information in the consent form than those who are ambulant. (Cassileth, B.R. *et al.*, 1980) Perhaps, as patients become more ill, their dependence on doctors increase and they have less interest in the consent form. It seems possible that comprehensive consent forms, designed for legal purposes, may in practice act as a barrier to 'true' informed consent.

It is not easy for patients with incurable cancer to make choices about treatment. As the chance of cure decreases, there may be a temptation to try more dangerous treatments with the risk of side effects, considerably lowering the quality of life. Often it is the patients who 'grasp at straws' and request such treatment. (Slevin, M.L. *et al.*, 1990)

There is no formula or figure which tells a surgeon that a choice of chemotherapy or operation is appropriate for a particular patient. He is guided by his clinical judgement, which is a personal perspective based on his clinical experience. Care should be taken to remember the patient's perspective and to offer alternatives and discuss choices. This 'sharing' option is clinically and emotionally more demanding for doctors, involves more time and a sensitivity to the ever-changing needs of the patient.

The act of informing is in itself a powerful sign of respect for the patient's autonomy. The doctor's aim should be that 'medical' choices that a patient makes should be no less informed than any other important decision they make in their lives. It is for patients to decide too, how much information is necessary. Doctors should be aware that patients who initially say that 'doctors know best' may be too confused or frightened to make a decision. They may wish to be helpful, or feel grateful, nor not want to be seen as 'trouble makers'. (Phillips, M. *et al.* 1985) Part of a doctor's skill is to see beyond the brave face and to explore the real needs and wishes of the dying patient.

A patient may choose not to be informed. Such a waiver of informed consent does not mean that the patient is giving up his rights to information in the future. It does constitute a valid consent even if it is not an informed one. Doctors should ensure that the 'waiver' is genuine and not just accept it as a practical short cut to obtaining informed consent.

Obtaining informed consent may be time-consuming and therefore consideration must be given to the costs to other patients. Information and knowledge not only improve patient morale but create trust; without open and honest communication, trust between doctor and patient evaporates. Because ultimately we are never fully informed, voluntary or autonomous persons, it does not necessarily follow that we are never adequately informed, free and autonomous. (Beauchamps, J.L., Childress, J.E., 1983)

Informed consent in palliative care preserves the patient's dignity. This sharing acknowledges that the emotional feelings and social experiences of patients may play a more important role in influencing their decisions than do medical issues.

Research in Palliative Care

Patients who are no longer curable by standard treatments are vulnerable to exposure to new and untried treatments in clinical research trials. Alternatively, patients may demand an untested treatment which might have been hailed in the media as a breakthrough. Unless these treatments are subjected to research trials involving patients, doctors will continue to lack the scientific evidence to judge which are most effective. A natural dilemma exists between the doctor's duty to do the best for his individual patient and his responsibility to develop improved treatments for future care.

Informed consent can be a valuable mechanism for moderating the pace of scientific progress in order to show care and respect for patients. It means that progress will still be made with informed agreement from the patients, and ensures that the subjects of therapeutic research are treated as individuals and not merely 'as means to others' ends'.

The requirement for informed consent makes doctors more aware of the effects of their intervention and more accountable for their decisions. Obtaining informed consent from each and every patient is therefore essential if doctors are to meet appropriate standards of both clinical care and therapeutic research. Although it may be difficult to define when ordinary treatment ends and clinical research begins, patients should be informed if part of their treatment is involved in a clinical trial. (Gillon, R., 1989) The Randomised Clinical Trial (R.C.T.) is a tool which is widely used in clinical cancer research. Ethical problems arise because doctors have to admit that they do not know which is the best treatment for the particular patient. They have a duty also to inform the patient that their treatment will be decided by randomisation.

Doctors are faced with dilemmas: it is unethical to enrol a patient as a research subject in a R.C.T. if this will result in less effective for that patient, any R.C.T. involves at least the risk of sub-optimal patient care. It is also unethical to subject patients to untested treatments, which may be dangerous or useless as well wasteful of precious resources. Many patients are unaware of the high levels of uncertainty which often exist in medicine. If the patient has expressed preferences in fulfilling his part of the informed consent procedure, it is most unlikely that he or she will want to accept treatment chosen by a lottery.

In the treatment of breast cancer, for example, R.C.T.s are usually preceded by pilot studies, so it is likely that doctors will have pre-trial preferences. Some surgeons believe that lumpectomy is better than mastectomy, while others are convinced that mastectomy is the treatment of choice. All of these may be reluctant to relinquish their decision-making power and to admit uncertainty. For the doctor to enter a patient in a R.C.T., a balance of expected benefit must exist between the standard and the trial treatment. The doctor may assure the patient that what is being offered is the best known treatment, since before the trial is completed there is no scientifically validated evidence that one treatment is better than another.

Scientific validation holds when results are 95 per cent certain. The patient may not be aware of this statistical convention, or that it may conceal underlying value judgements which they may not share. (Schaffer, A., 1989) It seems reasonable for patients to expect doctors to share their treatment preferences even when these fall below a confidence level of 95 per cent.

The research situation is complicated further by the fact that during the course of R.C.T. a trend may emerge favouring one therapy over and above another. The doctor's responsibility is to communicate these trends to patients to fulfill his obligation in informed consent. The patient should be free to withdraw from a trial at any stage if he chooses. One means of dealing with the problem of 'gradually arising news' would be for a different group of doctors to have access to interim trial results, not making these results available to the doctors involved in treating the patients. Merely involving more people, however, does not dilute the moral issue of withholding relevant information from patients. (Schaffer, A. 1989) If randomisation is too problematic or embarrassing for doctors to explain to patients, then it is randomisation that should be sacrificed, not the truth. (Faulder, C., 1985)

'Informed consent' in summary

It has proved consistently difficult to devise informed consent practices which satisfy, in full, the moral requirements of respect for autonomy, beneficence and justice. Sometimes these principles compete and doctors are faced with the dilemma of striking an ethical balance.

Informed consent protects patient autonomy, thus factors which ensure truly informed consent enhance autonomy. Time and privacy contribute to an environment where patients can receive information and understand their options. Verbal communication is vital if true informed consent is to be achieved. It is necessary for doctors to check the level of the patient's understanding. The consent form should be signed and witnessed only after the patient has had adequate time to study it and given the opportunity to ask questions. (Simes, *et al.*, 1986) Trained nursing staff can play a useful role in answering questions and making sure the patient understands. The patient and family may be seen together by the doctor and the nurse.

In clinical research, informed consent plays an important part in setting standards of appropriate medical and nursing care. It could be instructive for doctors involved in research trials to consider how willing they would be themselves to be members of a R.C.T. group. Patients should know when they are involved in R.C.T.s, and that their treatment is not dependant upon agreeing to participate in research. If, in palliative care, a scientific enquiry conflicts in any way with patient autonomy, the highest priority should be given to the latter. The dignity and wishes of the dying patient should be the doctor's first concern.

Informed consent has wider implications in health care: by discussing issues of consent, the public become involved in decision-making and consequently better informed about cancer therapy and research. (Downie, R.S. *et al.*, 1987) Current guidelines on research consent do not incorporate any penalties for doctors who choose to disregard them. Experience in the USA has shown that complex, comprehensive consent forms designed to protect doctors may act as yet another barrier to informed consent. Ethical committees can help to improve documentation and thus help to achieve the goals of informed consent. These committees should take great care not to isolate medical ethics as an academic discipline for intellectual debate, but to bring ethics to the bedside, where a personalised approach is the appropriate model of care.

All professionals should appreciate that informed consent is not a tiresome procedure which conforms to some bureaucratic demand but an integral element of respect for the patient. Indeed, the term 'informed consent' is too narrow and suggests the formality of obtaining a signed document. It represents a far wider concept, the importance of which should be acknowledged by referring to it as 'free, informed and understood consent.'

Chapter 7

Euthanasia: The Limits of Respect for Autonomy

A patient's request for assistance in ending his or her life presents the doctor with a moral challenge to his training and medical ethos. If respect for the patient's autonomy has the highest priority in ethical palliative care, the limits to this respect require exploration in order to help doctors determine their response.

Recently there has been increased interest in the moral arguments surrounding euthanasia. (Anon, 1992; Dyer, C. 1992) A British Medical Association report concluded that euthanasia was 'intuitively wrong'. (B.M.A. Working Party, 1988) Subsequently, a working party of the Institute of Medical Ethics suggested that 'assisted death' should be acceptable in certain clinical situations. (IME, 1990) The debate is fuelled by a medical technology which allows death to be postponed and increases patient life expectation, at the same time as there are limited financial resources for health care. Equally, some patients have become wary of medical technology which may also allow a prolonged undignified process of dying, and this has raised interest in the patient's 'right to die'. These issues will be explored here with reference to a case study.

Mrs. C.

Mrs. C., a terminally ill woman with advanced breast cancer, was in severe pain. She knew there was no possibility of cure and asked her general practitioner if he would help her to die by giving her a massive dose of tranquillisers. He refused her request and arranged her admission to hospital. The doctor in the ward explained that he could control her pain by using a continuous slow injection of a strong analgesic (Diamorphine) by a syringe pump which was changed every twenty-four hours.

A few days later, Mrs. C. was visited by her son who was a medical student. He was shocked and deeply distressed by the marked deterioration in his mother's physical condition. During his visit, his mother begged him to end her suffering. While the nurses were out of the ward, he injected the entire contents of the twenty-four hour syringe in a single dose.

Shortly after he left, his mother was found in a coma by a nurse. Noticing that the syringe pump was empty, the nurse immediately resuscitated Mrs. C. The son was arrested on a charge of attempted murder. One week later his mother developed a bronchopneumonia but was not given antibiotics. She died a day later, from the chest infection. The son was tried and discharged by the court.

Euthanasia literally means 'a good death' but the word has acquired different interpretations, the major one of which implies the positive attempt to end the life of a patient. The son who attempted to kill his mother by giving her a large injection was intending active euthanasia. Because it was requested by his mother, it is known as active voluntary euthanasia, or 'assisted death'. This is direct contrast to 'involuntary euthanasia' where the patient does not wish death or assistance at that stage. In withholding antibiotics for the bronchopneumonia, the doctors were refraining from treating a potentially remediable condition which resulted in the death of the patient, and this inaction is described as 'passive euthanasia'. Passive euthanasia may involve withholding necessary effective treatment, physically neglecting the basic needs of the patient such as food and water, or as in the above case, taking a decision not to prescribe futile treatment as the patient approaches death. (Wilkinson, J. 1990)

The Patient

'A patient's sustained wish to die is a sufficient reason for a doctor to allow him to do so.' (*Institute of Medical Ethics,* 1991)

Referring to the case study of Mrs. C., it is of importance to examine the reason why this patient requested active voluntary euthanasia. She was suffering severe pain which prompted her to make the request. It could be argued that if palliative care was improved, and pain controlled, requests for euthanasia would be eliminated, or rightly be regarded as irrational. (Parker, M., 1990)

Second to the level of pain being experienced by the patient, comes the question as to whether or not doctors are qualified to judge that this 'suffering' is always a negative value. Indications are that patients demonstrating endurance in spite of pain, have enriched the lives of their families and their carers. The process of dying is different for each individual, and may be a time of personal growth, even though some stages may be painful. For some a dignified death is a quiet, painless process but others 'rage against the dying of the light'. (Thomas, D., 1982)

The possibility should be considered that even if her pain was relieved, the patient might still have requested euthanasia. Arguments about the adequacy of palliative care do not reveal anything about the morality or the meaning of the request for euthanasia, and how in any particular case, the request is to be interpreted. Mrs. C.'s suffering may have been exacerbated by a feeling that she was burdening others. Her request for assistance may have been a test to see if others still valued her life. In refusing her request and sending her to hospital, the general practitioner may have been rejecting her 'cry for help' which could have been a veiled attempt to gain extra support to enable her to remain in her own home.

Any terminally ill patient may be vulnerable to subtle pressure from the family to request active euthanasia. Economic pressures could also tempt some doctors and health service managers to favour euthanasia as a cheaper, practical solution to the expensive problem of caring for the terminally ill. It is difficult for the professionals being asked to assist in 'a good death' to determine the blend of selfish and unselfish motivations lying behind the patient's request.

Mrs. C. may have felt that as she no longer had control, the only way of exercising her autonomy was to choose to die, and to do so sooner, rather than later. Respect for autonomy however, carries the limitation that such respect does not infringe the autonomy of others. In this case, Mrs. C.'s request interfered with the autonomy of the general practitioner. Furthermore, exercising autonomy implies taking responsibility for one's decisions. Such a decision for Mrs. C. would have been for her to take her own life. By requesting her doctor's assistance to kill her, she is avoiding moral responsibility and was thus not acting in a truly autonomous way.

Patients with cancer may become clinically depressed. In such a situation feelings of low self esteem and suicidal ideas are common. Cancer is an illness which tends to isolate patients, and in that isolation a quick death may seem the best option. It is rather alarming to note that doctors often miss a diagnosis of depressive illness, particularly in the elderly. (Conwell, Y., 1991) If a doctor is unable to recognise treatable depression then his response to a depressed patient's request for assisted suicide may be based on his own fears about ageing, cancer and dependency. Physicians may underestimate the remediable element of depressive illness. The whole concept of 'rational suicide' remains controversial.

The fact that the patient has a depressive illness does not necessarily mean that the choice he makes is irrational, any more than the absence of mental illness implies that decisions are therefore rational. Consideration has to be given to how severe depression must be before it precludes rational decision-making. The patient may not be clinically depressed, but 'appropriately' distressed and shocked by the predicament being faced. Though there is no general 'rule of thumb' that can be followed, doctors should concentrate on helping patients to think as rationally as possible in these situations. Many professionals lack these specialised psychiatric skills: without these skills and an awareness of their importance, doctors may agree to 'assisted death' when appropriate psychiatric treatment might change the patient's choices.

Respecting patients' autonomy means recognising that dying patients can still make choices. The terminally ill individual requires time to come to terms with symptoms, to assess the past and to find meanings. The choosing of active euthanasia, however, precludes all these choices, thus limiting autonomy. Since the time span regarded as 'terminal' is variable, there is no way of predicting for certain when death will take place. Killing someone two months before they would have died might be regarded as active, voluntary euthanasia, whereas two years before, would probably be termed murder. Death with dignity is hard to define because the perception of indignity often lies with the observer. The moral challenge for doctors is to see that the life of a wasted, jaundiced, dying patient is still of infinite value. Devaluing and/or not supporting such a life on the basis of age, non-productivity, cost or degree of physical handicap is not morally acceptable.

In spite of Mrs. C.'s request for euthanasia she was resuscitated by the nurse. Some patients have made written directives known as 'living wills' or advance directives, which state the wish not to be resuscitated in certain clinical situations, e.g., advanced cancer or dementia. A living will is the name which has been adopted for a document which allows a 'competent person to request and direct that certain measures be taken should he become incapable of taking responsibility for his own health care'. (Greaves, D. 1989) Living wills have no legal force in Britain but are legal in some parts of the USA. Medical practice in the USA is more interventionist than in Britain, especially in relation to continuation of life-sustaining treatment. Living wills (or advance directives), nonetheless, are not a substitute for good communication between patients and doctors. The honest approach is to take steps to elicit the patient's choice in a sensitive manner and to record this information, then to communicate it to the rest of the team. Improved communication would do much to calm the anxieties of patients about unnecessary treatments and lead to a reduced demand for living wills. Living wills also do not take into account the fact that patients may wish to change their minds during the course of their illness.

There are no cultural norms or agreements as to what should be done in these situations. It is difficult to draft a living will that is flexible enough to reflect even an individual's wishes. The presence of a living will may be of some help in influencing a doctor's decisions, but it is a sad reflection on the quality of the doctor-patient relationship, that a resort to such a device is considered necessary in palliative care.

The patient may argue that if free choice is said to be respected by the medical profession, should it not also be respected when the choice has to be made as to death or life? There is in fact a difference between the 'right to die' and the right to be assisted in dying. When a patient makes an autonomous choice of suicide then there is no criminal offence. (*Suicide Act*, 1961) Assisting in suicide, however, remains an offence under criminal law. It may seem illogical that to assist a person to perform a non-criminal act, is itself a crime. However, the attitude reflected in the law, is that killing in this sense of assisted suicide, or assisted death, should be considered as murder. In practice, however, the law recognises the necessity of allowing mitigating circumstances and in the case of Mrs. C., the son was discharged by the court.

The law clearly prohibits all actions causing intentional death. The Suicide Act , in legalising suicide, was a pragmatic response to the practical problem of administering sanctions to suicide victims rather than acknowleding the 'right to die'. In prohibiting killing, the law acknowledges the 'sanctity' of life and ensures that any 'right to die' cannot be a 'right to kill'.

Judaeo-Christian values emphasise the 'sanctity of human life'. This doctrine reflects the view that all human life is of infinite and intrinsic value and prohibits shortening of life. Hence, if human life can be prolonged, it is the doctor's duty to do so. Euthanasia is necessarily final and it removes any chance for the patient to revoke choices made.

The Medical View

British Medical Association guidelines and legal advice indicate clearly that active euthanasia is unacceptable and against the law. (BMA, 1988) There is a strong legal and moral prohibition against killing in our society, and there is no legal right for a person to authorise another to kill him. Killing is not permitted except in cases of self-defence, just war, or capital punishment, and even these circumstances are hotly debated. In none of these situations is the killing for the benefit of the person killed, but is allowable only to protect the lives or welfare of others. (Callahan,D., 1989)

The sanctity of life doctrine, for doctors, is emphasised in the Hippocratic Oath. Part of the essential qualification of being a doctor is an absolute rejection of killing the patient. A patient's trust and expectation of doctors as healers is based on this premise. Doctors have special duties of beneficence and non-maleficence; to kill a patient is to override both of these duties. It is likely that many patients might be deterred from seeking medical advice, if a part of the doctor's role was to kill patients (even if upon request). A natural outcome might be to lead patients to conceal symptoms lest doctors decided their lives were no longer 'worthwhile'.

Many of the arguments against active voluntary euthanasia take the form of a 'slippery slope' argument. This is to infer that if doctors were to allow active voluntary euthanasia in certain specific circumstances, it would mean a generalised 'stepping on the slope' which could lead in imperceptible steps to involuntary euthanasia. The slope could be one which reduces the physicians' sensitivities to killing, then slackening their professional resolve to save and prolong life. (Crispell, K.R. *et al.*, 1987) These arguments against active voluntary euthanasia stiffly maintain a psychological barrier against killing and allow no erosion of this principle. Such views preclude any moral change, even in cases of potential assisted death of those incapable of physically commiting suicide. Perhaps a more ethically-based principle than this broad prohibition would be to consider a case by case analysis. Otherwise, it could be inferred that there are limits to the kinds of question which should be raised in philosophical debate. What is required is sensitive, moral argument in each clinical situation.

The act of active voluntary euthanasia is final and makes no allowance for mistaken diagnosis. There is the concern that a diagnosis of terminal illness can be extended to include any medical condition which would result in death if treatment was no longer continued. Such a definition would include many insulin-dependent diabetics. The fact that there is a strong prohibition on active euthanasia has, in part, driven the improvements which have occurred in the care of the dying in the last twenty years.

It is surprising that a working party of the Institute of Medical Ethics concluded in a majority view that, 'a doctor acting in good conscience is ethically justified in assisting death if the need to relieve intense and unceasing pain or distress caused by an incurable illness, greatly outweighs the benefit to the patient of further prolonging his life'. (IME,

1990) The hospital doctor, in the case study, took a decision not to treat the episode of bronchopneumonia and this allowed Mrs. C. to die through a process of passive euthanasia. The doctor argued that there is a moral difference between killing and letting die. Passive euthanasia is merely an extension of good medical care. In this case it was withholding futile treatment of a life-threatening chest infection, because Mrs. C. had advanced cancer and was likely to die in the next few days. Although allowing the patient to die may seem less wrong than deliberate killing, the moral judgement should take account of the intention of the doctor, the circumstances and the consequences of the act, despite the fact that the outcome of active and passive euthanasia may be the same: the death of the patient.

The traditional medical view that it is worse to kill than to let die, reflects the Acts and Omission Doctrine derived from Roman Catholic theology. The doctrine argues that actions that result in some undesirable consequence are morally worse than a failure to act which has the same consequence. Foot gives an example: it is worse to send starving children in Africa parcels of poisoned food, than refraining from sending a cheque to Oxfam, though the consequence of either act or omission will be that children will die. (Foot, P., 1980)

Rachels presents a counter-example from which he maintains that the 'bare difference' between acts and omissions is not necessarily significant. (Rachels, J., 1986) Smith and Jones both stand to inherit a fortune if their six year old cousin predeceases them. Smith drowns his cousin in the bath making it look like an accident. Jones intends drowning his cousin but on entering the bathroom sees the boy fall and slide unconscious into the water. Jones waits to see that the boy dies and does nothing to help him. Rachels argues that both Smith and Jones are equally culpable and that in the absence of other morally important difference, the 'bare difference' between acts and omission, between killing and letting die is not itself morally significant.

Rachels' argument is that there is no necessary moral difference between killing and letting die, if other things are equal. In clinical practice, however, other things are seldom, if ever equal, and so one cannot state that killings are necessarily morally equivalent to letting die. (Gillon, R., 1988)

If a doctor kills a patient to save his ward budget, that action is morally wrong. Yet allowing the same patient to die at her request from a chest infection which is treatable, may be morally right. Doctors owe patients a duty not to kill them, but feel less strongly that they have to 'strive officiously to keep alive'. (Clough, Arthur Henry cited in Glover, J., 1977) Respect for autonomy may be thought to have little influence on the moral difference between killing and letting die, but this is not the truth. If the hospital doctor continued to treat Mrs. C. who had already expressed a wish to die, this would be failing to respect her autonomy. Refusing to kill her does not infringe that same autonomy as her own right to kill herself has not been withdrawn. Withholding life-prolonging antibiotics, in this case, was not only morally permissible but morally required. Doctors should not be required to promote life-prolonging treatments without regard for the patient's wishes.

Intuition tells us that if we kill someone we are the cause of the death, but by letting that person die, the death is derived from the chest infection or the cancer. It could be argued that the doctor had a special duty to Mrs. C. and that he has 'acted' in deciding not to treat. The danger of this argument is that we may fail to recognise the world external to the self, i.e. that the doctors do not control everything both within and outside the self. The reality of the disease cannot be overlooked. To withhold antibiotics from Mrs. C. may or may not be morally acceptable, but this does not alter the practical reality that the physical cause of death was widespread cancer with a consequent pneumonia. Doctors are not obliged to struggle endlessly to resist the lethal power of disease if a patient is unwilling to have it resisted, or where resistance no longer serves the patient's welfare.

Roman Catholic theology claims that not only is the outcome of a person's action important in a moral analysis, but also the person's intentions and obligations. (Linacre Centre, 1987) Intended consequences are distinguished from those unintended, the principle of double effect. Thus the doctor giving a slow injection of morphine with the intention of relieving pain, is not morally culpable, if a side effect was that the patient developed a fatal bronchopneumonia. It is diffcult, nonetheless, to clearly distinguish what may be foreseen as a side effect from an intention.

Another theological doctrine, relevant to the debate, is that of ordinary and extraordinary means. The statement is that the good of saving life is morally obligatory if its pursuit is not excessively burdensome or disproportionate to the expected benefit. (Gillon, R., 1989) Ordinary means are morally obligatory, such as food and water, extraordinary means are morally optional. There are, however, no clear boundaries between ordinary and extraordinary, i.e. is it ordinary or extraordinary to give antibiotics? The burdensome quality of treatment has to be determined in each individual case. The patient's interests are the prime moral concern.

In the case of Mrs. C. it is not clear that antibiotics would be an extraordinary treatment, but this decision was made in light of the futility of treatment in the individual case. Hence, a judgement about desirability of treatment must be made in advance of the judgement on what is 'excessive treatment'. The result is that thoughts about ordinariness or extraordinariness are of no help in decisions on whether or not a treatment should be given.

Philosophical analysis of the intuitive component of a doctor's judgement is difficult. The distinction between active and passive euthanasia is sometimes morally important and sometimes not, depending on the case. Since each case must be considered individually, attempting to make an overall moral distinction between killing and letting die may not be a useful exercise for patients or professionals. The doctor may be convinced that there is a significant moral difference, and this conviction arises from the central moral dictum of the ultimate sanctity of life. When 'quality of life' issues are raised, active euthanasia becomes a possibility, but nevertheless a weighty burden on the sensibilities and intuitive feelings of the caring professions.

The General Practitioner's 'gut feelings' were against active euthanasia for Mrs. C. and his intuitive response was to refuse her request. This refusal, however, was his own value judgement and cannot be taken to imply that all doctors would have shared similar views. It is possible that if the terminally ill themselves were 'polled', their own views on active voluntary euthanasia would differ from those of healthy people, including doctors. Clinical experience in hospice medicine reveals that requests from patients for euthanasia are rare events. The counter to this observation, made by those advocating euthanasia, argues that within the hospice environment, patients may not feel free to make such requests.

We should recognise and take account of the bond of trust developed between the general practitioner and the patient in the years when treatment was given with curative intent. (Roy, D. 1987) There may be a tendency to view this emotional relationship as obstructive in a moral analysis because it exposes the doctor's vulnerability. But, the emotions, values and intuitions of the doctor have to play a part in the relationship with the patient, therefore must be taken into account in any moral analysis.

British medical practice can be contrasted with that in Holland, where active voluntary euthanasia is carried out within certain guidelines. (Rigter, H. *et al.*, 1988) Doctors working within the guidelines are not legally prosecuted but abuses of the system do occur. (Fenigsen, R., 1989) In some cases, doctors have tried to coerce patients to undergo voluntary euthanasia. The existence of the choice for active euthanasia puts the elderly and terminally ill under some pressure to choose this alternative. Fenigsen alleges, that not only is voluntary euthanasia common in Holland, but there is widespread public support for 'involuntary' euthanasia. This form of involuntary euthanasia, sometimes described as 'crypthanasia', enjoys judicial leniency in Holland. Crypthanasia is resorted to when doctors find it difficult to talk openly to patients about active euthanasia. This difficulty in itself throws doubt on the voluntary nature of voluntary euthanasia, and would seem to offer further argument for rejecting active euthanasia altogether.

The Son of Mrs. C.

Mr. C.'s prime motive was compassion for his mother's distress. He responded to her request by trying to give her a quick, painless death. An appeal to compassion does not alter the legality of the wrong but it does modify the moral position. Mr. C. had been informed that his mother was dying, and prolonging the suffering was unnecessary.

The son might back his argument with evidence of popular support for active voluntary euthanasia (Rigter, 1988) but the morality of euthanasia cannot be determined on the basis of an opinion poll. Public opinion is often unreliable because it is susceptible to emotive manipulation by the media. After a particularly tragic case the public might be moved to legalise euthanasia in the same way as the popular press demands a return to capital punishment after a horrifying murder.

Any change in the status quo related to euthanasia would, of course, require informed debate which would have to take account of public opinion. This is the discussion to which the British Medical Association and the Institute of Medical Ethics are contributing through their working party reports. There is also the need to isolate the primary moral debate from issues of health care resources devoted to care of the dying.

Little is said of the way assisted death is to be brought about, but some suggestions have been made that narcotics could be used. (IME, 1990) When Mr. C. injected all of the remaining diamorphine into his mother, his expectation was that she would die peacefully. Clinical practice has shown, however, that when a patient receives gradually increasing doses of diamorphine to relieve pain, it is unlikely to prove fatal. If narcotics are employed as tools of euthanasia, cancer patients may assume a doctor is suggesting euthanasia when he is employing morphine appropriately to relieve pain. Some patients are reluctant to receive such appropriate treatment for pain, fearing they will have an earlier death. Studies have shown the opposite, that when pain is well-controlled patients may live longer. (Twycross, R., 1991)

Mr. C. would also have been faced with a dilemma if he was opposed to euthanasia. He was distressed by his mother's suffering and he felt a duty to help at the same time as he did not want to kill her. His own autonomy was overridden by his duty to his mother, and he also had the problem of adjusting to his own loss. The grieving process often begins before death. He doesn't want her to die but feels her suffering is intolerable. His action in injecting the diamorphine is a measure of just how distressing it is for relatives to watch a loved one 'suffer'.

Perhaps, if the son had received support and help from a medical and nursing staff sensitive to his suffering, he might not have felt driven to his desperate act. In appropriate palliative care the needs of the family should receive just as much attention as those of the patient. The law in this case took account of these considerations in sentencing, and the son, accused of attempted murder, was discharged by the court. This decision was not a legal endorsement of active euthanasia, but a recognition of the extreme level of distress experienced by some relatives.

Nurses and euthanasia

The nurse is guided by the law which prohibits killing and by nursing codes of ethics. In Britain, the United Kingdom Central Council (UKCC) issues a code of conduct for the Nurse, Midwife and Health Visitor, stating that the nurse shall 'act always in such a way as to promote and safeguard the well-being and interests of patients'. (UKCC *Code of Conduct*, para. 1) Also, 'the nurse shall ensure that no action or omission on his/her part or within his/her sphere of influence is detrimental to the conditions or safety of patients'. (para. 2)

The nurse in the case study was presented with the dilemma of deciding whether or not to resuscitate a patient with advanced malignant disease. The dilemma existed partly because there was no clear decision made by the patient, her family, doctors or nurses. In the emergency situation the nurse's reaction was a 'paternalistic' one to institute resuscitation even though aware that Mrs. C. had requested euthanasia and had no wish to live. The nurse may be prompted by fears of litigation and censure by nurse management and medical colleagues. Aware that a crime had been committed, the nurse would be conscious that the case would be examined in the courts. In the hospital setting, in contrast to the patient's home, a large number of medical and nursing staff are involved in the care of a patient, and covert acts of active euthanasia are unlikely to happen without discovery.

Whether or not the doctors and nurses had discussed the question of resuscitation with Mrs. C., no record of a decision was made in the patient's notes. Now that patients have access to their notes, there may be a greater reluctance to record such decisions. While it could be suggested that the nurse, with prior knowledge of Mrs. C's wishes, violated her autonomy by resuscitating her, it is not for nurses to decide whether or not to resuscitate. Within their code of conduct they are obliged to preserve life unless there has been a medical decision, involving the patient and the family, that active resuscitation would be futile.

Appropriate Models of Care

Improved communication between doctors, nurses, patients and their families will lead to a better mutual understanding of the patient's wishes. Active euthanasia should be rejected, but patients should have symptoms controlled and their families supported. This type of balanced care can be given in a hospital or community setting, not only in hospices. 'Hospice' is a model of care not a building. Patients need the time of doctors and nurses to listen to their views. Treatment of cancer may have ceased but treatment of the patient carries on until the moment of death. Living wills are a symptom of society's fear of medicine's potential to 'overtreat' and are not a solution to the problem. If living wills are given legal status we will have taken a first step in the direction of legalising euthanasia. Killing is not morally acceptable but letting die may be different and acknowledges that death is a natural end to life.

The focus of care is the patient, but the professionals also need help and support. Decisions are sometimes difficult to make. Most doctors have been involved in the care of patients where active euthanasia would have been a possibility. At the same time, there is the realisation of the harms resulting from even a small erosion of the prohibition of killing. The medical profession has duties and obligations to aid the dying as autonomous and dignified individuals, and there is a qualitative difference between being a dispenser of death and a doctor who will help a patient in the difficult process of dying. (Miller, P.J., 1987) Whilst professionals need to examine carefully our motives for intervention, it is also incumbent on 'society' to reach agreements on the proper care of the dying. (Smith, R., 1992)

Euthanasia and allocation of resources to the dying are separate moral issues. (Crispell, K.R. et al., 1987) It is possible for many individuals to die at home with their families without the use of expensive 'high' technology, if they are well informed and allowed to express their own desires. Primarily this means listening to the views of patients expressed as they may be, in 'the common tongue', rather than couched in terms of ethical analysis. Caring based on sound moral principles is best achieved by doctors, nurses and other health care professionals communicating with each other and the patient, and working together as a team.

Chapter 8

An Ethical Model of Palliative Care

In this concluding chapter, a summary is given of an ethical model for the palliative care of patients who are struggling with, and dying of, incurable diseases. Palliative care aims to maximise the quality of life of a patient with incurable cancer. A number of ethical dilemmas arising in this context have been identified.

Respect for the patient's autonomy is proposed as having the highest priority in an ethical model of palliative care. To respect autonomy is to respect the whole person in the context of his relationships with other individuals and involves acknowledgement of the doctor's own emotions. For professionals to deny emotions and feelings of vulnerability in themselves, and in their patients, is to deny compassion, and to distance themselves from patients. (Alderson, P., 1991) Compassion is an essential part of the doctor-patient relationship and the health team-patient relationship.

Ethical frameworks based purely on abstract theories of deontology (the branch of ethics dealing with duties and moral obligations) or utilitarianism may seem far removed from the everyday clinical situation. Utilitarianism may seem to discriminate against the individual cancer patient, when care is directed toward ideas of doing the greatest good for the greatest number. The impersonal 'duties' related to deontological theory, however, may not be appropriate for the emotional aspects of the care of a patient who is suffering. Both of these theories place great emphasis on pure reasoning and seem to reflect a rejection and mistrust of emotions. These theories do not take account of the practical problems encountered in palliative care. Similarly, models based on the quartet of autonomy, beneficence, non-maleficence and justice are most useful in abstract analysis but less helpful in the setting of close relationships. (Gillon, R., 1985) (Beauchamp, T.L., Childress, J.E., 1983)

It has become evident in this study of palliative care that if an ethical framework is to be of practical use to patients and staff, respect for autonomy needs to be combined with a caring approach. Such a model has the advantage of acknowledging that feelings, compassions, integrity and virtue play a vital part in the holistic approach to care.

Medical ethics is not solely concerned with abstract arguments, but also with the practicalities of supporting patients who may be distressed. Sharing may involve both doctor and patient acknowledging their own vulnerability and limitations. A close moral relationship requires trust, compassion and involvement of both doctor and patient. Inequalities of power may act to prevent patients from expressing their views. Sharing involves listening to patients: the 'patient's voice' may not articulate views in ethical jargon, but these views are still morally valid and require attention. A partnership between the professional and patient acknowledges the differences in power but also recognises that all individuals have equal moral status.

Ethical decisions should be considered in the context of an individual clinical case and not only in abstract isolation. Clinical and ethical decision-making are closely linked; doctors should listen to their intuitive voice which tells against killing but permits letting die in certain situations. To permit doctors to kill patients at their request would be to damage their healing power and to increase the potential to dominate patients.

The ethical model which combines respect for autonomy with a caring ethos within the professional-patient partnership needs also to take account of the value of teamwork. A team approach allows health care professionals to share problems and to co-ordinate different skills for the benefit of the patient. There may be problems in reaching a moral consensus; clinical decision-making needs to be informed by medical ethicists and philosophers, who in turn need to be involved with patients and to hear the 'patient's voice' at first hand. The role of the ethicist is to unravel the ethical issues not to provide a 'right answer'.

The process of attempting to resolve ethical dilemmas may cause stress to doctors and nurses. There is a necessity for those working in palliative care to meet together for mutual support. In the process of identifying the ethical issues in palliative care, an ethical model of appropriate care has emerged. While recognising that each case should be considered in an individual way, it has been possible to derive an ethical framework to help health professionals to provide better palliative care. By highlighting the essential elements in the morally challenging relationship between one who is dying and the one and the many who are involved in that death.

¤ THE ETHICAL MODEL OF APPROPRIATE PALLIATIVE CARE

¤

RESPECT FOR AUTONOMY

- Avoiding 'strong' paternalism which threatens autonomy

- Adopting a broad approach to autonomy which permits 'weak' paternalism

- Sharing truthful information about diagnosis, treatment and prognosis with the patient, in a sensitive manner

- Presenting the patient with choices

- Seeking the patient's free, informed and understood consent

A CARING PARTNERSHIP

- A partnership between doctors, other health care professionals and the patient based on trust and an open honest approach

- A commitment to teamwork, a partnership between health carers

- A holistic approach to care

- Acknowledging uncertainty and vulnerability

- Listening to the patient

- Avoiding distancing, sharing emotional involvement and compassion with the patient and her family

A SHARED CULTURE

- Promoting the acceptance of death

- Resolving unfinished business

- Demystifying cancer and death

- Acknowledging the value of life and rejecting active euthanasia

- Accepting that 'letting die' may be permissible in some circumstances

- Making an appropriate transition between a curative and a palliative approach to care, with the patient's consent and comprehension

- Taking account of the patient's view on the quality of his or her life

CARE FOR THE CARERS

- Supporting the patient's family

- Supporting doctors and nurses and other health care professionals

- Recognising and avoiding burn-out

¤

Appropriate palliative care demands that the medical team combine respect for the patient's autonomy with a caring morality. This involves a partnership with the patient. In this relationship moral dilemmas are shared with compassion and humility to the mutual benefit of the professional and the patient. By employing this ethical model in the care of patients with incurable cancer, at no time should the professional feel: 'There is nothing more I can do'.

Bibliography and references

Abbreviations

AIM Annals of Internal Medicine

BMA British Medical Association

BMJ British Medical Journal

BME Bulletin of Medical Ethics

IME Institute of Medical Ethics

JME Journal of Medical Ethics

New Eng.J.Med. New England Journal of Medicine

Aitken, H. (1991) Someone to turn to, *BMJ* 302: 185.

Alderson, P. (1991) Abstract bioethics ignores human emotions, *BME* May:13-21.

Anon. (1968) Research without consent continues in the U.K., *IME Bulletin,* July:13.

Anon. (1992) The final autonomy, *Lancet* 340:757-758.

Appelbaum, P.S., Grisso, T. (1988) Assessing the patient's capacities to consent to treatment. *New Eng.J.Med.* 319: 1635-8.

Ashby, M., Stofell, B. (1991) Therapeutic ratio and defined phases: proposal of an ethical framework for palliative care, *BMJ* 302:1322-4.

Baum, M., Zilkha,K., Houghton, J. (1989) Ethics of clinical research: lessons for the future, *BMJ* 299:251-3.

Beauchamp, T.L., Childress, J.E. (1983) *Principles of Biomedical Ethics,* Oxford University Press.

Blyth, A.C. (1990) Audit of terminal care in a general practice, *BMJ* 300:983-6.

Boston, S., Trezise, R. (1987) *Merely Mortal,* Methuen.

Brett, A.S. (1988) 'The patient's expectations in the United States' in *Cost versus Benefit in Cancer Care* : 39-49, Stoll, B.A. (Ed.), Macmillan.

BMA Working Party (1988) Euthanasia, *BMJ* 296:1376-7.

Buckman, R. (1984) Breaking bad news. Why is it still so difficult?, *BMJ* 288:1597-9.

Callahan, D. (1989) Can we return death to disease?, *Mercy, Murder and Morality: Perspectives on Euthanasia:* 4-6, Hastings Center Report.

Calman, K.C. (1984) Quality of life in cancer patients - an hypothesis, *JME* 10:124-7.

Cassileth, B.R., Zupkis, R.V., Sutton-Smith, K., March, V. (1980) Information and participation preferences among cancer patients. *AIM* 92:832-6.

Cassileth, B.R., Luck, E.J., Strouse, T.B., Bodenheimer, B.J. (1984) Contemporary, unorthodox treatments in cancer medicine, *AIM* 101:105-112.

Clough, A.H. (1977) 'The latest decalogue', cited in Glover, J., *Causing Death and Saving Lives*, Penguin.

Conwell, Y., Caine, E.D. (1991) Rational suicide and the right to die, Reality and myth, *New Eng.J.Med.* 325:1100-3.

Crispell, K.R., Comez, C.F. (1987) Proper care of the dying: a critical public issue, *JME*, 13:74-80.

Daly, M.E. (1987) Towards a phenomenology of caregiving: growth in the caregiver is a vital component, *JME*, 13:34-9.

Daniels, N. (1986) Why saying no to patients in the United States is so hard, *New Eng.J.Med.* 314:1380-3.

Degner, L.F., Russell, C.A. (1988) Preferences for treatment control among adults with cancer, *Research in Nursing and Health*, 11:367-74.

Downie, R.S., Calman, K.C. (1987) *Healthy Respect*, Faber & Faber.

Dworkin, G. (1972) Paternalism, *Monist* 56:64-84.

Dworkin, G. (1988) *The Theory and Practice of Autonomy*, Cambridge University Press.

Dyer, C. (1992) Rheumatologist convicted of attempted murder. *BMJ* 305:731.

Edelwich, J., Brodsky, A. (1980) *Burn-out: Stages of disillusionment in the helping professions,* Springer, N.Y.

Fallowfield, L.J., Baum, M. (1989) Psychological welfare of patients with breast cancer, *Journal of the Royal Society of Medicine* 82:4-5.

Farsides, C.C.S. (1989) It's a hard life bein' a guinea pig - The problems of human experimentation, in *By what right? Studies in Medicine, Ethics and Law*:35-52, P. de Cruz, McNaughton, D. (Eds.).

Faulder, C. (1985) *Whose body is it?* Virago Press.

Fenigsen, R. (1989) The case against Dutch Euthanasia, *Mercy, Murder and Morality: Perspectives on Euthanasia*:22-30, Hastings Center Report.

Firth-Cozens, J. (1987) Emotional distress in junior hospital doctors, *BMJ* 295:533-6.

Field, D. (1989) *Nursing the Dying,* Tavistock/Routledge.

Foot, P. (1980) The problem of abortion and the doctrine of double effect: 156-65, in *Killing and Letting Die,* Steinboch,B. (Ed.), Prentice-Hall.

Ford, G.R., Pincherle, G. (1978) Arrangements for terminal care in the NHS, *Health Trends* 10:73-6.

Fottrell, E. (1990) Multidisciplinary functioning: will it be of use? *British Journal of Hospital Medicine* 43:253.

Gillett, G.R. (1989) Informed consent and moral integrity, *JME* 15:117-23.

Gillon, R. (1985) *Philosophical Medical Ethics* John Wiley.

(1988) Living wills, powers of attorney and medical practice, *JME* 14:59-60.

(1989) Deciding not to resuscitate, *JME* 15:171-2.

(1989) Medical treatment, medical research and informed consent, *JME* 15:3-5.

(1990) Deceit, principles and philosophical medical ethics, *JME* 16:59-60.

Girad, M. (1988) Technical expertise as an ethical form: towards an ethics of distance, *JME* 14:25-30.

Gough, I.R., Furnival, C.M., Schilder, L., Grove, W. (1983) Assessment of quality of life of patients with advanced cancer, *European Journal of Cancer,* 19:1161-5.

Greaves, D. (1989) The future prospect for living wills, *JME* 15:179-82.

Greer, S. (1983) Cancer and the mind, *British Journal of Psychiatry* 143:535-43.

Griffin, J. (1991) *Dying with dignity,* Office of Health Economics, No. 97.

Harris, J. (1987) QALYfying the value of life, *JME* 13:117-23.

Hinton, J. (1979) Comparison of places and policies for terminal care, *Lancet* 1:29-32.

Independent, The (1991) Cuts force rethink on cancer treatment, 18 May:1.

IME (1990) *Viewpoint: Assisted death,* Working party on the ethics of prolonging life and assisting death, Lancet 336:610-3.

Jolley, M.G. (1988) Ethics of cancer management from the patient's perspective, *JME* 14:188-90.

Kearsley, J.H. (1986) Cytotoxic chemotherapy for common adult malignancies: "the emperor's new clothes" revisited? *BMJ* 302:1-2.

(1989) Compromising between quantity and quality of life, in *Ethical Dilemmas in Cancer Care,* Stoll, B.A. (Ed.), Macmillan.

Klein, R. (1991) On the Oregon trail: rationing of health care, *BMJ* 302:1-2.

Kubler-Ross, E. (1970) *On Death and Dying,* Tavistock.

Lamb, D. (1990) A plea for a touch of idealism: reply to P. Whitaker, *JME* 16:134-5.

Lichter, I. (1987) *Communication in Cancer Care,* Churchill Livingstone.

(1989) The right to bad news, in *Ethical Dilemmas in Cancer Care*, Stoll, B.A. (Ed.), Macmillan.

Linacre Center (1978) *Is there a morally significant difference between killing and letting die?* London.

Lovestone, S., Fahy, T. (1991) Psychological factors in breast cancer, *BMJ* 302:1219-20.

Maguire, P. (1985) Barriers to psychological care of the dying, *BMJ* 291:1711-13.

Maguire, P., Faulkner, A. (1988) How to improve the counselling skills of doctors and nurses in cancer cases, *BMJ* 297:847-9.

(1988) Communicate with cancer patients: 1, Handling bad news and difficult questions, *BMJ* 297:907-9.

(1988) Communicate with cancer patients: 2, Handling uncertainty, collusion and denial, *BMJ* 297:973-4

Millar, P.J. (1987) Death with dignity and the right to die: sometimes doctors have a duty to hasten death, *JME,* 13:81-5.

Mooney, G. (1989) QALYs: are they enough? A health economist's perspective, *JME* 15:148-52.

Nash, A. (1989) A terminal case? Burnout in palliative care, *Professional Nurse,* June:443-4.

Palmer, B.V., Walsh, G.A., McKinna, J.A., Greening, W.P. (1980) Adjuvant chemotherapy for breast cancer: side effects and quality of life, *BMJ* 281:1594-7.

Parker, M. (1990) Moral intuition, good deaths and ordinary medical practitioners, *JME* 16:28-34.

Phillips, M., Dawson, J. (1985) *Doctors' Dilemmas,* Harvester Wheatsheaf.

Rachels, J. (1986) *The End of Life: Euthanasia and morality*, Oxford University Press.

Rees, G.J. (1985) Cost-effectiveness in oncology, *Lancet* 11:1405-7.

(1991) Cancer treatment: deciding what we can afford, *BMJ* 302:799-800.

Reynolds, M. (1978) No news is bad news: patient's views about communication in hospital, *BMJ* 1:1673-6.

Righter, H., Borst-Eilers, E., Leenon, H.J.J. (1988) Euthanasia across the North Sea, *BMJ* 297:1593.

Roy, D.J. (1987) Ethics in palliative care, *Journal of Palliative Care,* 3:1.

Saunders, C. (Ed.) (1984) *The Management of Terminal Malignant Disease,* Edward Arnold: 1-9.

Schafer, A. (1989) Achieving informed consent in clinical trials, in *Ethical Dilemmas in Cancer Care*, Stoll, B.A. (Ed.) Macmillan.

Searle, C. (1991) Communication and awareness about death: a study of a random sample of dying people, *Social Science Medicine* 32:943-952.

Simes, R., Tattersall, M.H.N., Coates, A.S., Raghauan, D., Solomon, H.J., Smart, T. (1986) Randomised comparison of procedures for obtaining informed consent in clinical trials of treatment for cancer, *BMJ* 293:1065-8.

Slevin, M.L. (1992) Quality of life: philosophical question or clinical reality?, *BMJ* 305:466-9.

Slevin, M.L., Plant, H., Lynch, D., Drinkwater, J., Gregory, W.M. (1988) Who should measure the quality of life, the doctor or the patient? *British Journal of Cancer*, 57:109-12.

Slevin, M.L., Stubbs, L., Plant, H.J., Wilson, P., Gregory, W.M., Armes, P.J., Downer, S.M. (1990) Attitudes to chemotherapy: comparing views of patients with cancer with those of doctors, nurses, and the general public, *BMJ* 300:1458-60.

Smith, R. (1992) Euthanasia: time for a royal commission. *BMJ* 305:728-729.

Sontag, S. (1979) *Illness as Metaphor,* Penguin.

Spiegel, D., Kraemer, H.C., Bloom, J.R., Cottheil, E. (1989) The effect of psychological treatment on survival of patients with metastatic breast cancer, *Lancet* Oct. 14:888.

Stoll, B.A. (1990) Choosing between cancer patients, *JME* 16:71-4.

Suicide Act, Acts of Parliament, United Kingdom (1961)

Sutherland, H.J., Llewellyn-Thomas, H.A., Lockwood, G.A., Tritchler, D.L., Till, J.E. (1989) Cancer patients: their desire for information and participation in treatment decisions. *Journal of the Royal Society of Medicine* 82:260-3.

Thomas, D. (1982) From 'Do not go gentle into that good night' cited in *The Rattle Bag*, Heaney, S., Hughes, T. (Eds.) Faber & Faber, London.

Townsend, J., Frank, A.O., Fermont, D., Dyer, S., Karran, O., Walgrave, A., Piper, M. (1990) Terminal cancer care and patients' preference for place of death: a prospective study, *BMJ* 301:415-7.

Twycross, R. (1990) Viewpoint: Assisted Death: a Reply, *Lancet* Sept. 29:796.

United Kingdom Central Council (UKCC), *Code of Professional Conduct for the Nurse, Midwife and Health Visitor* (1984) Para. 1.2.

Vachon, M.L.S. (1987) Battle fatigue in hospice/palliative care, International Symposium on Pain Control. *Royal Society of Medicine International Congress and Symposium Series*, No. 123:69-75.

Veatch, R.M. (1989) *Death, Dying and the Biological Revolution,* Yale University Press, New Haven & London.

Wanzer, S.H., Adelstein, S.J., Craford, R.E., Federman, D.D., Hook, E.D., Moertel, C.G., Safar, P., Stone, A., Taussig, H.B., Vane, Y.S. (1984) The physician's responsibility towards hopelessly ill patients, *New Eng.J.Med.* 310:955-9.

Wilkinson, J. (1990) The ethics of euthanasia, *Palliative Medicine* 4:81-6.

Wilson-Barnett, J. (1989) Limited autonomy and partnership: professional relationships in health care, *JME* 15:12-6.

INDEX